ISBN: 1478262303
ISBN 13: 9781478262305

Thank you . . .

To Debbie, my wife now of more than thirty-eight years, for helping and supporting me all those years with my management of diabetes!

To my parents, Sidney and Maxine, for helping me to accept responsibility for my health with diabetes, beginning in the first grade and for all the encouragement you gave!

THE WAY OF WISDOM FOR DIABETES

Cope with Stress, Move More,
Lose Weight and Keep Hope Alive

KEN ELLIS

Contents

Introduction

The Way of Wisdom for Diabetes Self-Management

Would you like to hear words that build your confidence, words that are positive and uplifting, words that are motivational, words that give you a greater sense of hope for better health and well-being? I believe we would all like to hear words like that, wouldn't we? Then read this: *"Wisdom is sweet to your soul; if you find it, there is a future hope for you, and your hope will not be cut off"* (Proverbs 24:13).

Read the following words and see if they also give you a greater sense of hope and confidence: *"Accept what I say. Then you will live for many years....Listen closely to my words....They are life to those who find them. They are health to your whole body....For through wisdom your days will be many, and years will be added to your life. If you are wise, your wisdom will reward you....Having respect for the LORD leads to a longer life"* (Proverbs 4:10, 20, 22, 9:11–12, 10:27). If you've read those words in the book of Proverbs before, did they grab your attention, alerting you to the fact that they can directly be applied to handling diabetes or any chronic disease? It's a rare commentary on Proverbs that relates these words to your physical wellness. Well, there is much more helpful information to learn for health and wellness, and it is called *wisdom! Wisdom* is skill for living. *"A good person gives life to others; the wise person teaches others how to live"* (Proverbs 11:30). *"Those who get wisdom love their own lives; those who cherish understanding will soon prosper"* (Proverbs 19:8).

The Road to Good Health Is Always under Construction. When You Are Through Learning, You Are Through. Keep Learning!

We all are susceptible to falling into the trap of thinking we know more than we actually do. None of us wants to be like the person who had diabetes for twenty years, but had stopped learning after the first year. Sure, that person may have accumulated twenty years of "hard knocks" experience, but the experience will be more difficult, with diabetes complications, if learning and applying is not continually done! Blood glucose monitors, the glycemic index, "feel full on fewer calories" strategies, and A1c tests were management techniques unheard of several years ago. Newer, more accurate information is available today! That is why we need to keep learning! I like the following humorous saying; it shows a vivid picture of what happens when we become closed-minded and stop learning:

Don't be so narrow-minded that your ears rub together.

Knowledge is better than feelings. Ever tried just going by your feelings to determine where your blood sugar really is? I've been caught off guard at times, thinking I have a low blood sugar level, when in reality it's high. You can feel hunger pangs when you are high as well as when you are low. To see how accurate your feelings are, estimate what your number will be before you even check your blood sugar. I lived for twenty years with diabetes before glucose meters were even available. During those years it would have been nice to check the feelings of hunger or weakness with a glucose meter. Some people, however, who have had diabetes a number of years can experience low blood sugar unawareness. That is another reason why it is important to check blood sugar levels, instead of guessing.

There is always more to learn. Did you know that some people, who are newly diagnosed and are at the beginning stages of Type 2 diabetes don't have to be on medications to increase the level of insulin to experience low blood sugar? A newly diagnosed person came to me experiencing low blood sugar. How could this even happen without being on any medications? Did you know that one of the first symptoms of Type 2 diabetes is to lose phase one of insulin release? A certain messenger (a hormone, GLP-1) comes from the small intestine to the pancreas, signaling for insulin to be released, because the person has eaten some carbohydrates. There is no insulin to release, so in phase two, production starts. As a result, in trying to catch up with the needs to metabolize the food, more insulin may be produced than is needed, resulting in a low blood sugar a few hours later.[1] So we need to keep learning—it is our responsibility to do so! *"The way of a foolish person seems right to him. But a wise person listens to advice"* (Proverbs 12:15).

The Best Helping Hand You Will Find Is at the End of Your Own Arm

---

Several years ago a photographer from a well-known national magazine was assigned to cover the fires at Yellowstone National Park. The magazine wanted to show some of the heroic work of the firefighters as they battled the blaze.

When the photographer arrived, he realized the smoke was so thick that it would seriously impede or make it impossible for him to photograph anything from the ground. He requested permission to rent a plane and take photos from the air. His request was approved, and arrangements were made. He was told to report to a nearby airport, where a plane would be waiting for him.

He arrived at the airport and saw a plane warming up near the gate. He jumped in with his bag and shouted, "Let's go!" The pilot swung the little plane into the wind, and within minutes they were in the air.

The photographer said, "Fly over the park and make two or three low passes, so I can take some pictures."

"Why?" asked the pilot.

"Because I am a photographer," he responded, "and photographers take photographs." The pilot was silent for a moment. Finally he stammered, "You mean you're not the flight instructor?"

When it comes to your diabetes, who is the pilot? Ultimately it has to be the person with the diabetes. We do, however, need good information by which to pilot our decisions; and ultimately we have to implement what we learn. As soon as we accept that responsibility, realizing that the greatest ability we have is the ability to respond (responsibility), we'll be set free to outsmart diabetes. Jack Paar said, "Looking back, my life seems like one long obstacle race, with me as the chief obstacle." D. L. Moody wrote, "I have had more trouble with myself than with any other man." We can relate to what they have said, because when it comes to managing diabetes, we can be the obstacle. We all need to realize that we can ultimately be in control. It is like what Dr. Gary Arsham wrote: "You are the best available source of support for living well with diabetes. You are always there and you know yourself well; no one else can take care of you as well as you can."[2]

The Way of Wisdom: The Proverbs

In accepting personal responsibility, the factor that is usually not included for navigating safely over, around, and through diabetes obstacles is the way of wisdom. In this book, I want to introduce, for your use, God's powerful provisions through his wisdom. *"I guide you in the way of wisdom. I lead you along straight paths. When you walk, nothing will slow you down. When you run, you won't trip and fall. Hold on to my teaching. Don't let it go. Guard it well. It is your life"* (Proverbs 4:11–13).

It is really interesting that his wisdom states that *"If you are wise, your wisdom will reward you"* (Proverbs 9:12). One of the rewards is usually better health and wellness. *"They are the key to life for those who find them; they bring health to the whole body"* (Proverbs 4:22).

When people accept the responsibility to take care of their bodies, they usually end up feeling better! *"Those who find me find life, and the Lord will be pleased with them. Those who do not find me hurt themselves. Those who hate me love death"* (Proverbs 8:35–36).

Fundamentals: The Human Body, with Proper Care, Will Last a Lifetime
---

These wisdom teachings of Proverbs are fundamentals. They are the basic guidelines and patterns for living well. It doesn't make sense to talk about new fundamentals. That's like saying someone has made some new antiques. It is a contradiction in terms. Since they are brief, basic principles that need to be mastered for healthy living, they don't deal with exceptions to their guidelines. For example, we assume that at a red traffic light, people will stop, but there are exceptions to the rule. So these wisdom fundamentals are not a guarantee that you will live longer, but an observation of what usually happens. In that sense, they are promises for health and wellness!

Gems or Nuggets

The way of wisdom, or proverbs, have been described as gems that have been cut and polished to such a high degree that they display a dazzling splendor. They give an image or a picture of life or reality. With short, pithy, descriptive comparisons they make the basic truths they portray easier to remember and use. In fact, the word that is translated proverb basically means "to be like," "to resemble," or "to represent."

On the surface, we may think we understand the full meaning of a proverb, but when we ponder and examine it more carefully, we discover even more richness in meaning. It is like a light going through a prism and coming out on the other side, with the rich colors of a rainbow. To illustrate this, notice how the example of an ant is used in Proverbs 30:25 - *"Ants are creatures of little strength, yet they store up their food in the summer."* The obvious meaning is to save your money for the future. When this is done, it will alleviate much stress in a person's life. To effectively cope with stress is a major factor for maintaining good health. I'll examine the hidden factor of stress on blood sugar control in chapter 8.

When we dig deeper, however, we discover another application that directly relates to the health of our whole bodies. How do ants store up their food? They do it by constantly being on the move. And movement is the application to our diabetes self-management, which I'll examine in detail in chapter 11.

Also ants are said to have "little strength." Besides being on the move to gather their food, they also work together! One person, while walking, noticed "a vast army of ants carrying an earthworm. It was so startling that I stopped to watch the action. The earthworm—shaped more or less like a treble clef—appeared to have dried out in the sun. All around the earthworm were ants, pushing away. And they were moving it one micro-inch at a time. I didn't count, but I would bet there were at least fifty ants pushing away at that poor dead earthworm. All around them were other ants, several hundred of them, 'junior varsity' ants waiting for their chance to get in the game."[3] One ant couldn't have moved the earthworm by itself, but with the help of dozens of ants the earthworm was being moved. To be wise like an ant means we support each other. When we face the challenge of a chronic disease like diabetes, it is best to face it with the help and encouragement of others! And that is the relevance to our health and wellness that I will explore in chapter 7. So *"Go to the ant . . . consider its ways and be wise! It has no commander, no overseer or ruler, yet it stores its provisions in summer and gathers its food at harvest"* (Proverbs 6:6–8).

The Proverbs Are Timeless and Time-Tested

The Proverbs are supported by the experience and observations of generations of wise people. These individual proverbs, which are often just two lines, have been described as "compressed experience." Many of them are attributed to King Solomon, but many of them are also called "the sayings of the wise." These proverbs go beyond mere human experience; they also are endorsed by God.[4] I'm writing about this in the hope that these fundamental principles for living will provide hope, strength, and a compelling motivation for you to put them into practice! They can help us all to cope with the challenges we face with diabetes. They will also give us greater success to triumph over a disease that is seemingly harmless, but can be very dangerous because it is too often underrated! Even though there are now many new resources available for the management of diabetes, they still won't work if we're not motivated to consistently use them. People need an unfailing, empowering aid to implement these resources, and that is what the *"Way of Wisdom"* will do!

"Don't be wise in your own eyes. Have respect for the LORD and avoid evil. That will bring health to your body. It will make your bones strong" (Proverbs 3:7–8).

---

1. Richard Beaser, MD, ed., *Joslin Diabetes Deskbook: A Guide for Primary Care Providers* (Boston: Joslin Diabetes Center, 2010), 5, 168, 212.
2. Gary Arsham, MD, and Ernest Lowe, *Diabetes: A Guide to Living Well* (Alexandria, Virginia: American Diabetes Association, 2004), 15.
3. Ray Pritchard, *The ABC'S of Wisdom: Building Character with Solomon* (Chicago: Moody Press, 1997), 68-69.
4. James E. Smith, *The Wisdom Literature and Psalms* (Joplin, Missouri: College Press Publishing Company, 1996), 464–67.

Part 1

Staying Motivated To Do The
Things We Need To Do

Chapter 1

Keeping Hope Alive, Fighting Off Discouragement

When I was diagnosed on December 20, 1960, with Type 1 Diabetes, I was in the first grade, and the little word *diabetes* had such an impact on my dad that he became lightheaded and almost passed out. I'm sure that reaction has been exhibited numerous times by other parents of children with diabetes. Anyone, however, who hears the words "You have diabetes," whether it is Type 1 or Type 2, will be hearing three words he or she doesn't want to hear!

In fact, to hear "You have diabetes" can even be a devastating blow to some people. Why is that? *Change*, *fear*, *shame*, and *denial* are words that come to mind. Often people who hear those words 'have known others with the disease—like an uncle or aunt, mother or father, cousin, or friend—and the complications they experienced with it. It can be scary, and they dread experiencing the same things. Another reaction can be denial. They just won't accept the diagnosis and stubbornly refuse to follow the guidelines given. They may also begin to dread the changes that have been recommended for them to make! Hope is needed, whenever difficult circumstances are faced.

A good example of what hope can do is well illustrated in the following story. A boy was in the hospital, suffering from severe burns. Obviously, he was not able to be at school. A large school district was using volunteers to tutor children who were forced to miss school due to illness. A woman who had volunteered for this service was given the following instructions from this boy's teacher: "We're studying nouns and adverbs in his class now, and I'd be grateful if you could help him understand them, so he doesn't fall too far behind."

When the woman arrived at the hospital room, she found the young boy lying on the bed in great pain. Overwhelmed by the sight of this boy, all she could do was blurt out, "I've been sent by your school to help you with nouns and adverbs." After working with the child for a time, she left, feeling foolish. What good were grammar lessons to a boy in his condition?

However, her visit had a tremendous impact on the boy. Before seeing the tutor, the boy had been slowly deteriorating. After her visit, he seemed to find his will to live, working with therapists, eating meals, and responding to treatments. Later the boy explained, "I had just about given up, assuming I was going to die. But when this teacher came, I realized that I was going to be all right. They wouldn't send someone to work on nouns and adverbs with a dying boy, would they?"

What this woman shared about grammar was of minimal benefit to the boy, but the hope she brought to his life made all the difference. Hope saved his life. Paul writes to *"rejoice in hope"* (Romans 12:12). *"For everything that was written in the past was written to teach us, so that through endurance and the encouragement of the Scriptures we might have hope"* (Romans 15:4).

Many doctors, parents, and friends have always known how important it is to give hope to people. Dr. Elliott Joslin tried to give hope even before the discovery of insulin. The Joslin Diabetes Center in Boston, which is affiliated with Harvard Medical School, was named after him. He specialized in the treatment of those with diabetes for almost thirty years before insulin was discovered in 1921, and another forty years after it was discovered. Another doctor, Seale Harris, expresses what both of them saw, especially in children with Type 1 diabetes before the discovery of insulin in 1921: "I treated diabetics for twenty-nine years before Banting and his confreres gave us insulin, and I saw many patients die after a few months or a few years of semi-starvation. The children and the coma cases always died. Even now

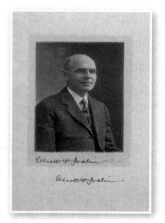

I do not like to recall the feeling of hopelessness I felt when diabetics came for treatment and the many sad scenes I witnessed which the use of insulin would have prevented."[1]

Dr. Joslin wrote about those early days before 1921, when there was no insulin, and the prognosis of children. He said, "That tender-hearted parents sometimes ask, and sympathetic friends nearly always ask: 'Since diabetes is always fatal in children, why prolong the agony? Why not let the poor child eat and be happy while life lasts?'" He gave the following

Dr. E. P. Joslin of Boston was one of the first doctors to receive insulin for his patients. Photo courtesy of The Thomas Fisher Rare Book Library, University of Toronto.

5

two reasons for using the starvation to live longer therapy: first, "the mother must not be forgotten, and we cannot do her the injury of killing hope, of admitting, 'Yes, popular belief is true: your child can never grow up.'" The second reason he gave to not give up was that "courage has lengthened the lives of many diabetic children, and no man knows but that the cure may be at hand within the year—even the month."[2] And sure enough, insulin was discovered, which prolonged the lives by decades of many people, including two individuals whose cases we'll examine: Elizabeth Hughes and James Havens. From their examples, 'we'll learn important life-changing applications.

Stay Motivated for Just One Day and Repeat That Day for a Lifetime!

Why focus on hope so much? A 2008 newspaper article's title was "Diabetes: Underrated, Insidious and Deadly."[3] It's underrated, people think, when compared to other conditions like cancer and heart disease. It's insidious or seemingly harmless because initially elevated blood sugars are doing their harmful work inside the body on organs and nerves unnoticed! It's deadly, because it puts people at a higher risk for heart disease and stroke and, as a result, death. The 2011 Diabetes Fact Sheet from the Centers for Disease Control states that diabetes is the leading cause of blindness for people age twenty to seventy-four and a leading cause of kidney failure and non-traumatic amputations. Sixty to 70 percent of people with diabetes have nervous system disease—neuropathy. Someone might counter those facts by saying that actually, it is "poorly controlled" diabetes that can cause those complications, not just diabetes. Control, however, is not a simple task; in fact, that's the big challenge—to find the motivation to stay in control!

A person has to stay motivated. Is it inevitable that 'you'll get complications if you're diagnosed with diabetes? No, complications aren't inevitable, if you can maintain your motivation—and not for just a day, but for a lifetime. So I'm writing this book to help you stay motivated each day. There have been many suggestions on how to do this, like linking a challenging activity with one that's fun and easy. For example, you could exercise and then reward yourself by watching your favorite TV show, or watch it while you walk on a treadmill, or exercise by walking with a friend.

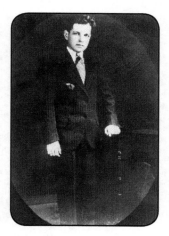

When insulin was discovered, the first person to receive a large, unrefined dose was a fourteen-year-old boy named Leonard Thompson. He had lived for two years on the "under-nutrition, starvation" therapy, which we'll review in the next chapter. He lived another fifteen years on insulin injections but was described as not a very well-controlled diabetic. His own behavior contributed to his deterioration and death.[4]

Leonard Thompson first person given insulin. Photo courtesy of Eli Lilly and Company Archives.

On the other hand, Teddy Ryder was five years old and weighed twenty-six pounds when he received his first dose of insulin. Dr. Banting, the discoverer of insulin, was the one who administered it. When Teddy's uncle, Dr. Mortin Ryder, asked for insulin for his nephew in the summer of 1922, Dr. Banting suggested that he write again in September. The supply was too unstable or impure to use. Dr. Ryder replied, "Teddy won't be alive in September."

So, Dr. Banting decided to accept him as a patient. Teddy was a person who had loving people who cared about him and from whom he learned to be motivated to take care of himself. He lived for seventy years with daily insulin injections. He died in 1993 at the age of seventy-six, the last of the original group of Dr. Banting's patients.[5] Again, motivation is key!

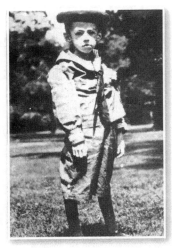

Teddy Ryder before insulin. Photo courtesy of Eli Lilly and Company Archives.

"Every Day Can Be Tough, but When the Water Starts to Rise, So Can You!"

The Browns were shown into the dentist's office, where Mr. Brown made it clear he was in a big hurry. "No fancy stuff, Doctor," he ordered. "No gas or needles or any of that stuff. Just pull the tooth and get it over with."

"I wish more of my patients were as stoic as you," said the dentist admiringly. "Now, which tooth is it?"

Mr. Brown turned to his wife. "Show him, honey." It's easy to be brave, strong, and motivated when you're not the one in pain!

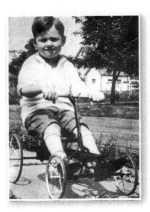

Teddy Ryder one year after taking insulin. Photo courtesy of Eli Lilly and Company Archives..

It's also easy for someone to say, "You need to check your blood sugars at least twice a day, lose fifty pounds, eat a balanced meal, and walk four miles a day." It puts me in mind of my doctor, almost forty years ago, telling me I wasn't taking care of myself. He said, "When you first came to see me, you didn't even know what you were eating or how much you were eating." He told me to take better care of myself while he smugly sat behind his desk, smoking a cigar.

We can learn from those living with diabetes how "Every Day Can Be Tough!" You may also be able to relate to some of the challenges some have expressed that make each day tough—challenges like the ones listed below.

Daily Tasks: "It's all the tasks one must do each day." "It's remembering to take your medications each day at the proper time." "It's a full-time job that nobody gets paid for." "It's something you wake up with and go to bed with every day. In other words, there is no vacation from diabetes." "It's avoiding certain kinds of food that will directly affect your blood sugar levels."

Low Blood Sugars (Hypoglycemia): "It's coping with the anxiety that comes from low blood sugars and properly handling the lows when they come. Just dealing with lows can disrupt the day, leaving a person exhausted."

The Unexpected: "It's the struggle with keeping blood sugars in a normal range, especially when eating out." "Spontaneous activities can present a real challenge with low blood sugars. For example, when you just took your insulin for a meal, and friends ask you to take an unplanned walk after the meal."

Complications from High Blood Sugars: "It's facing the complications and discomfort that high blood sugars bring to your feet—painful neuropathy." "High blood sugars also result in becoming dehydrated, having no energy, and repeated trips to the restroom."

The Simplicity of Diabetes Management?

Diabetes management may seem simple. After all, all I have to do is take my insulin at the right time, in just the right amount, several times each day; check my blood sugars multiple times a day to make sure I'm not too high or too low; balance the right amount of food with the insulin I take; and move frequently throughout the day. Stay alert at all times, just in case something goes wrong. And also realize this must be done every day, because there is never a vacation from diabetes. That's how simple it can be!

After reading those challenges, we can all relate to how important motivation is. One common factor for motivation is hope, and the source of hope that is commonly overlooked is God's wisdom. Listen to these words from the book of Proverbs: *"Eat honey, my son, for it is good; honey from the comb is sweet to your taste. Know also that wisdom is sweet to your soul. If you find it there is a future hope for you and your hope will not be cut off"* (Proverbs 24:13–14). Notice what gives hope? It is wisdom! Wisdom is the skill for living and is needed for health and wellness.

Do You Desire to Live a Longer Life?

It would be easy for a person newly diagnosed with diabetes to express thoughts like the following:

"I feel overwhelmed," or "I have so much to learn and understand," and "I don't know if I can do things right."

Instead of having those discouraging thoughts, why not focus on the following words from God's wisdom, words like: "*Through me, you will live a long time. Years will be added to your life. If you are wise, your wisdom will reward you*" (Proverbs 9:11–12). "*My son, do not forget my teaching, but keep my commands in your heart, for they will prolong your life many years and bring you peace*" (Proverbs 3:1–2).

The apostle Paul also wrote about staying motivated and not giving up. The principles he teaches are also seen in the wisdom principles listed in the book of Proverbs. Notice the following guidelines that apply to not giving up, staying motivated, and staying in control. The fundamental teachings will also apply to diabetes management.

Look on the Brighter Side of Life: Be Thankful.

"*...be prepared to **endure everything** with patience, **while joyfully giving thanks** to the Father*" (Colossians 1:11–12). Here, persevering goes hand in glove with giving thanks. When we focus on what is good, the natural response should be to be thankful. According to Proverbs 15:30, focusing on the good news brings health to one's life: "*Good news gives health to your body.*"

Have Hope: A Confident Expectation That You Can Manage Diabetes.

"*...your **endurance inspired by hope** in our Lord Jesus Christ*" (1 Thessalonians 1:3). Paul specifically states that hope in Jesus keeps one from giving up, but don't overlook the basic principle that hope inspires endurance. According to Proverbs 24:14, a person has hope when wisdom is found, and that hope will remain with the person who finds it, inspiring a person to not give up. It says, *"Wisdom is sweet to your soul. If you find it, there is a future hope for you, and your hope will not be cut off."*

Be an Encourager: Encourage Others and You'll Be Encouraged.

---

*"So I **put up with** everything (or **endure** everything) for the good of God's chosen people..."* (2 Timothy 2:10). When a person's focus is on helping others, it also helps him or her to keep on keeping on when facing difficult times. According to Proverbs 11:25, when a person helps others, the help not only benefits others, it also uplifts the one giving the encouragement. *"A generous person will prosper; whoever refreshes others will be refreshed"* (Proverbs 11:25). *"A good person gives life to others; the wise person teaches others how to live"* (Proverbs 11:30).

Having had diabetes now for more than five decades, I've learned we must stay motivated and outsmart diabetes! We cannot just sit back, thinking that complications can come to others but not us. We can manage diabetes by using medical information and guidelines. The hidden factor for this achievement, though, which is usually not acknowledged, is again God's way of wisdom, the Proverbs.

They can empower you, motivate you, and give you hope. This wisdom was initially applied to managing my diabetes more than fifty years ago by my parents. I then learned to apply the principles myself. Notice what is stated in Proverbs 4:20–22: *"My son, pay attention to what I say; listen closely to my words. Do not let them out of your sight, keep them within your heart; for they* are life to those who find them and health to a man's whole body." Nine of those principles are listed below and will be explained in greater detail in the following chapters.

SOME OF THE "WAY OF WISDOM" PRINCIPLES ARE...

The Road to Good Health Is Always under Construction. When You Are Through Learning, You Are Through. Keep Learning!

"Those who cherish understanding will soon prosper" (Proverbs 19:8). "When pride comes, then comes disgrace, but with humility comes wisdom" (Proverbs 11:2). "The heart of the discerning acquires knowledge; the ears of the wise seek it out" (Proverbs 18:15). "A wise man has great power, and a man of knowledge increases strength" (Proverbs 24:5). "For waging war you need guidance, and for victory many advisers" (Proverbs 24:6). "If you falter in times of trouble, how small is your strength" (Proverbs 24:10).

Proper Prior Planning Prevents Pitifully Poor Performance. People Don't Plan to Fail, They Fail to Plan. Planning the Best Decisions Ahead of Time: Diligence

"The sluggard craves and gets nothing, but the desires of the diligent are fully satisfied" (Proverbs 13:4). "The wisdom of the prudent is to give thought to their ways, but the folly of fools is deception" (Proverbs 14:8). "A sluggard does not plow in season; so at harvest time he looks but finds nothing" (Proverbs 20:4). "The plans of the diligent lead to profit as surely as haste leads to *poverty"* (Proverbs 21:5). The basic meaning of diligence is planning ahead, which I'll review in chapter 12.

Don't Just Sit There, Keep Moving

---

*"Go to the ant, you sluggard; consider its ways and be wise! It has no commander, no overseer or ruler, yet it **stores** its provisions in summer and gathers its food at harvest"* (Proverbs 6:6–8). *"From the fruit of his lips a man is filled with good things, as surely as the **work of his hands** rewards him"* (Proverbs 12:14). *"All **hard work** pays off. But if all you do is talk, you will be poor"* (Proverbs 14:23). *"Ants are creatures of little strength, yet **they store up** their food in the summer"* (Proverbs 30:25). Keep in mind that when these proverbs were written most work involved manual labor.

Wise People Keep Themselves Under Control: Portion Control, Healthy Choices, and Self-Control

---

"If you find honey, eat just enough. If you eat too much of it, you will throw up" (Proverbs 25:16). *"It is not good to eat too much honey, nor does it bring you honor to brag about yourself"* (Proverbs 25:27). *"Like a city whose walls are broken through is a person who lacks self-control"* (Proverbs 25:28). *"Wise people see danger and go to a safe place. But childish people keep going and suffer for it"* (Proverbs 22:3). *"A fool gives full vent to his anger, but a wise man keeps himself under control"* (Proverbs 29:11).

Keep Working Patiently on the Small Stuff, Because Life Has a Way of Accumulating

---

"Dishonest money dwindles away, but he who gathers money little by little makes it grow" (Proverbs 13:11). *"Those who are patient have great understanding, but the quick-tempered display folly"* (Proverbs 14:29). *"With patience you can convince a ruler, and a gentle word can get through to the hard-headed"* (Proverbs 25:15).

Know the Condition of Your Health and Life. Keep a Daily Personal Health Inventory

---

"Be sure you know the condition of your flocks, give careful attention to your herds; for riches do not endure forever, and a crown is not secure for all generations" (Proverbs 27:23–24). *"There is a way that appears to be right, but in the end it leads to death"* (Proverbs 14:12). *"A simple man believes anything, but a prudent man gives thought to his steps"* (Proverbs 14:15). *"The best food and olive oil are stored up in the houses of wise people. But a foolish man eats up everything he has"* (Proverbs 21:20). *"Wicked people are stubborn, but good people think carefully about what they do"* (Proverbs 21:29).

Instead of Putting People in Their Place, Put Yourself in Their Place. Lift People Up, Don't Put People Down. If Discouraged, Encourage!

"A generous person will prosper; whoever refreshes others will be refreshed" (Proverbs 11:25). *"A good person gives life to others; the wise person teaches others how to live"* (Proverbs 11:30). *"A friend loves at all times. He is there to help when trouble comes"* (Proverbs 17:17). *"A generous man will himself be blessed, for he shares*

his food with the poor" (Proverbs 22:9). "As iron sharpens iron, so one person sharpens another" (Proverbs 27:17).

Be Careful What You Think, Because Your Thoughts Run Your Life! Have Positive Expectations of Yourself.

"As he thinks in his heart, so is he" (Proverbs 23:7). "Be careful what you think, because your thoughts run your life" (Proverbs 4:23). "Pleasant words are like honey. They are sweet to the spirit and bring healing to the body" (Proverbs 16:24). "The tongue has the power of life and death, and those who love it will eat its fruit" (Proverbs 18:21). "The right word spoken at the right time is as beautiful as gold apples in a silver bowl" (Proverbs 25:11).

Count Your Blessings, and You Will Show a Profit. Have the Attitude of Gratitude. Look on the Brighter Side of Life—The Good News.

"He who seeks good finds goodwill, but evil comes to him who searches for it" (Proverbs 11:27). "A happy heart makes the face cheerful, but heartache crushes the spirit" (Proverbs 15:13). "All the days of the oppressed are wretched, but the cheerful heart has a continual feast" (Proverbs 15:15). "A cheerful look brings joy to your heart. And good news gives health to your body" (Proverbs 15:30). "A cheerful heart makes you healthy. But a broken spirit dries you up" (Proverbs 17:22). "Hearing good news from a land far away is like drinking cold water when you are tired" (Proverbs 25:25).

When is the best time to learn these Biblical wisdom principles to help us avoid many physical ailments—and cope more effectively with those we must face?

I like the attitude of Cato the elder. He was a Roman scholar who began to learn Greek when he was more than eighty years old. When asked why he was tackling such a difficult, arduous task at his age, he replied, "It is the earliest age I have left." I like that attitude, don't you? Today is the earliest age we all have left! Let's keep learning!

1. Seale Harris, MD, *Banting's Miracle: The Story of the Discoverer of Insulin* (Philadelphia: J. B. Lippincott Company, 1946), xi.

2. Chris Feudtner, MD, *Bittersweet: Diabetes, Insulin, and the Transformation of Illness* (Chapel Hill: The University of North Carolina Press, 2003), 206–207.

3. Tara Parker-Pope, "Diabetes: Underrated, Insidious and Deadly," *New York Times* (New York, NY), July 1, 2008, www.nytimes.com/2008/07/01/health/01well.html?_r=1&ref=science (Accessed June 21, 2012).

4. Michael Bliss, *The Discovery of Insulin* (Chicago: The University of Chicago Press, 1982), 112, 243.

5. Thea Cooper and Arthur Ainsberg, *Breakthrough: Elizabeth Hughes, the Discovery of Insulin, and the Making of a Medical Miracle* (New York: St. Martin's Press, 2010), 176, 243.

Chapter 2

Learning from the Past Experiences of Others to Take Advantage of Resources Available Today

How can we stay motivated? Someone says, "You need to be more positive."

"How can I do that?" you say.

"You can do that by working harder!"

"How can I do that?"

"You can do that by being more positive." It ends up being a vicious cycle. The way of wisdom teaches, *"As iron sharpens iron, so one person sharpens another"* (Proverbs 27:17).

The story is told of two cowboys and a Native American traveling on their horses in the old west. The two cowboys started talking about how famished they were, and how when they got to town they would go to the nearest café and get a steak with all the trimmings. They asked their friend if he was hungry too, and he just nodded that he wasn't. When they got to town, they stabled their horses, and all three went to the café. All three of them ordered steaks with all the trimmings, and when their dinners came, the Native American friend wolfed his down faster than either of the cowboys. He gobbled everything in sight.

Watching him with some amusement, one of his friends reminded him that less than an hour before, he had said he wasn't even hungry. So why was he shoveling it in now? "Not wise to be hungry then," he said. "No food." In other words, he had learned to be content with what he had or didn't have.

Today, in thinking about diabetes, we have a lot of resources for diabetes self-management, for which we can be thankful. Do we really realize how much we actually have? If we were to look back on the experiences of others in the past, who were trying to cope with diabetes, we would be shocked at how few resources they actually had. When we actually look back, we'll realize how abundantly blessed we really are today.

In my seminar, I give a visual of comparing the past with the present by showing a small portion of a picture and then asking the audience what it is. No one ever comes up with the answer. The picture is just a small portion of my Boston Terrier's forehead. Then I show the whole picture. It does make a difference when the whole picture is seen. It also helps to see the whole picture of how diabetes has been treated in the past, compared with how it is treated today.

Recognizing all that has changed will fortify our motivation and give us a greater appreciation for all that is available today for outsmarting and living well with diabetes! It will also give us a foundation for developing one of the most powerful of the wisdom principles for health and wellness: gratitude. Let's take a short history tour now of how diabetes has been treated through the years, including my more than fifty year history. We'll then look at the medical research and scientific studies that have been done on gratitude, and then apply the Biblical wisdom principle of gratitude to our own lives.

There can be confusion about what to eat and what not to eat by those who are newly diagnosed with diabetes. One man said, "My doctor told me about the importance of a healthy meal plan, which—as near as I can tell—means I'm only allowed to eat birdseed all day." Well, it was almost that way before 1921.

"Eat Less, Be Hungrier!"

Based on Dr. Frederick Allen's research, the state-of-the-art therapy, especially for those with Type 1 diabetes, was a restriction on food. In 1919, Dr. Frederick Allen published *Total Dietary Regulation in the Treatment of Diabetes*, citing exhaustive case records of seventy-six of the one hundred diabetes patients he observed. He basically advocated to patients to eat less and be hungrier!

This "under-nutrition, starvation therapy" could prolong a person's life by a few months or even a few years by basically starving him or her to death. Few patients or their parents could tolerate such restrictions on basic food needs. There were exceptions like James Havens, who lived for more than seven years on this therapy; and Elizabeth Hughes, who lived for four years until the advent of insulin therapy. They were both fortunate enough to live until insulin was discovered and received some of the limited amounts that were first available.

The treatment would start with an extremely low-carbohydrate diet and gradually be increased to the renal threshold, or the level of blood glucose above which the kidneys fail to reabsorb—and thus spill—glucose into urine. The renal threshold is about 180 mg/dl. What this meant for most people was living on a diet plan or "starvation therapy" of very little food per day. For the teenage Elizabeth Hughes, it meant living on about an average of eight hundred calories per day.

People on this therapy were described by Dr. Elliott Joslin with the first ten verses of Ezekiel 37, as the "Valley of

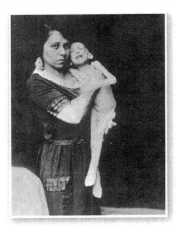

Three year old J. L. before insulin.
Photo courtesy of Eli Lilly and
Company Archives.

Dry Bones," referring to Ezekiel's description of the Jewish exiles from Judea to Babylon. "*Can these bones live?....I will cause breath to enter you so you will come to life. I will put muscles on you and flesh on you and cover you with skin. Then I will put breath in you so you will come to life*" (Ezekiel 37:1ff). These Jews were people who had everything taken from them—their homes, their way of life, their worship. They were taken hundreds of miles away without any future prospects of returning, of their lives turning back to how it used to be. They were in despair, without hope, and are described as just dry bones.

Hope, life, and well-being were gradually being taken from the patients that Dr. Joslin helped. He literally saw the "valley of dry bones" among these people with diabetes, who were gradually starving to death. In 1922, his description changed, because people were being restored to healthier life with the advent of insulin. One boy named J. L. weighed fifteen pounds on December 15, 1922, at the age of three, but after being on insulin for just two months, he weighed twenty-nine pounds. Dr. Joslin writes, "By Christmas of 1922, I had witnessed so many near resurrections that I realized I was seeing enacted before my eyes Ezekiel's vision of the valley of dry bones....It still remains a wonder that this limpid liquid (insulin) injected under the skin two times a day can metamorphosize a baby, child or frail adult

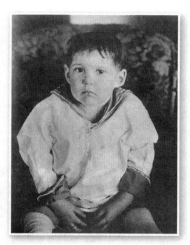

J.L. two months later, on insulin. Photo courtesy of Eli Lilly and Company Archives.

or old man or woman to their nearly normal counterparts."[1]

Dr. Frederick Allen's reaction was one of optimism for those under his care, after his visit to Dr. Banting in Toronto, Canada. Dr. Banting was a surgeon during World War 1. While in the battle zone, he was wounded with shrapnel in his right forearm. It was removed and a tourniquet was applied above his elbow. He then continued to work on the wounded for seventeen hours. This is the kind of character he had!

Dr. Frederick Banting and Charles Best discovered what came to be known as insulin on July 27, 1921. After his time in World War 1, he became a demonstrator in surgery and anatomy at the University of Western Ontario. It was in this role that he had to talk to medical students about the pancreas, which led him to read about the islets of Langerhans in a medical journal. From there he came up with an idea to extract a substance from

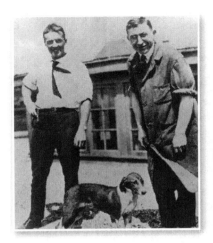

Charles Best and Dr. Frederick Banting, discoverers of insulin. Photo courtesy of Eli Lilly and Company Archives.

the islets, using the lab at Toronto University. He and a graduate student assistant, Charles Best, used the lab dogs, dog pound dogs, and even strays that summer for their experiments. They found what came to be known as insulin. The biochemist J. B. Collip refined the substance, and it was given to the first human recipient, fourteen-year-old Leonard Thompson on January 19, 1922, with spectacular results.[2]

Do You Know That You Have Some Very Small but Priceless Islands? The Islets of Langerhans

Today we know that each person has about one million of these islets in the pancreas. Each of these islets contains about two thousand beta cells and alpha cells (which manufacture the hormone glucagon). It is within the beta cells that insulin is manufactured in a multistep process. The word *insulin* is from a Latin root word meaning *island*. In Type 1 diabetes, these cells are rapidly destroyed, leaving nothing by which insulin can be produced. The beta cells also manufacture and store insulin that can quickly be deployed when carbohydrates are initially eaten. In Type 2 diabetes, that stored, first-phase insulin is often lost, and there can also be a resistance by the body's cells to the insulin that is produced.[3]

24

In 2010, my wife and I went to the Joslin Diabetes Center in Boston to participate in a research study called "The 50-Year Medalist Research Study." There have been about 750 people who have had diabetes for at least fifty years who participated in this study of Type 1 diabetes.

One important discovery the researchers have made is that two-thirds of the medalists still have a few beta cells in the pancreas, which can produce a very small amount of insulin. Forty percent of them have not developed any complications. The research is trying to determine how some of these cells have survived as well as to discover protective factors against complications. Even those who have the benefit of some insulin production are still dependent on daily injections of insulin.

The amount of insulin one produces can be determined by a test that measures c-peptides. When insulin is being produced, it comes from an A chain of fifty-one amino acids and a B chain of fifty-one amino acids that are brought together with connecting peptides, or c-peptide, until the insulin molecule is formed in a multi-step process.[4] In the final step of the process, the c-peptides are discarded into the blood, which can then be measured. In the test, they were looking for a range of 1 to 12 to determine insulin production. My wife, who was in the non-diabetes control group, had a 7.9, and mine was less than 0.05. In other words, my beta cells have been destroyed, which was originally thought to be the case for every person with Type 1 diabetes.

Another test we took showed the importance of insulin. We started the day fasting and when we got to the Joslin Diabetes Center they had me turn my pump off. Then we drank a flavored carbohydrate drink. It was similar to the oral glucose tolerance test, which contains about 75 grams of carbohydrate. My wife's level started at 79 fasting; then, after drinking the mixture, it was measured in thirty-minute intervals at 99, then 70, then 59, and after two hours 65. My test, without the benefit of insulin, went from 144 fasting to 207, then 260, then 329, and then after two hours 378. People without diabetes will usually maintain blood glucose levels below 120 mg/dl.

I Think We Have Something for You.

Dr. Frederick Allen visited Dr. Banting in Toronto on August 8, 1922. While he was away, rumors spread among his one hundred young patients at his clinic that something magnificent was about to happen for them. Before his return to his clinic, nurse Margate Kienast wrote: "...the mere illusion of new hope cajoled patient after patient into new life. Diabetics who had not been out of bed for weeks began to trail weakly about, clinging to walls and furniture....It was a resurrection, a crawling, stirring, as of some vague springtime." She continued, "Bed immediately after dinner was the rule for our patients. But not that evening.... When he appeared through the open doorway, he caught the full beseeching of a hundred pairs of eyes... his voice curiously mingling concern for his patients with an excitement that he tried his best not to betray...'I think,' he said, 'I think we have something for you.'"[5]

The discovery of insulin brought about dramatic changes and hope for a better life for those with diabetes. Today, many people with Type 2 diabetes may fear taking insulin, thinking their diabetes must be getting worse, injections will hurt, and they are nearing the end. "Insulin is just another tool for improved diabetes care—one of the most effective, in fact. It can actually improve your quality of life along with your diabetes control," writes Dr. Richard Jackson of the Joslin Diabetes Center.[6] All of this is actually good news, and the way of wisdom teaches, "*A cheerful look brings joy to the heart, and **good news** gives health to the bones*" (Proverbs 15:30). In addition to insulin, which has saved the lives of millions, there is now another tool that has brought dramatic improvements for those who meticulously use it.

Don't Test Your Blood Glucose Levels, Just Check Them!

A girl who was not quite four years old was alone in the house when the phone rang. Her mother was in the backyard. The little girl answered the phone and was told that Mr. Brown was calling, wanting to talk to her parents. She had seen her mother take messages, so she said, "I'm sorry, no one is here. Can I take a message?" After a pause, Mr. Brown heard, "OK, I'm ready. What was your name?"

"Mr. Brown."

"How do you spell Brown?"

"B-r-o-w-n."

A long pause, and then, "How do you make a B?" That is really getting back to fundamentals, isn't it? What is a fundamental for diabetes management? It is using a tool that lets you know what your current blood sugar level is. The tool, of course, is a blood glucose meter. By inserting a strip into the meter and then applying a small drop of blood to it, the result is displayed on a screen within five seconds.

It sounds so simple, doesn't it? Yet, many people neglect to use this tool. I was visiting with a couple in a doctor's waiting room, and we were talking about checking our blood glucose on a daily basis. He said his wife, who was sitting next to him, refused to do it on a regular basis. In fact, she hated to do it. I said I check myself about eight times a day. He asked, "How do you do that?" I said I just tell myself I love to check myself and do it. He told me to tell his wife that, and when I did, he said, "Preach on, brother, preach on." His wife's attitude is not uncommon!

There is a cartoon that says, "He's called Sir Lance-A-Lot, because he's always checking his blood glucose." Most people with diabetes couldn't have a name like that, because they simply don't check their blood glucose. An American Diabetes Association survey found that 21 percent of adults with Type 1 never check. Of those with insulin-treated Type 2 diabetes, 47 percent never check. Of those with Type 2 diabetes not using insulin, 76 percent never check.[7]

What makes it easier for me to check myself, which I've done now more than 95,000 times, is my gratitude for the blood glucose meter. Nothing like this was even available when I was first diagnosed in 1960. I lived with diabetes for twenty-one years before this tool even became available for my use.

What I used for twenty-one years was Tes-Tape, which is glucose analysis from the urine. The tape, when urine was applied, would change from yellow to a light, medium, or dark green, depending on how much glucose was present. Of course, this would not give a current reading, like checking blood glucose does today. Remember the renal threshold, or the level of blood glucose above which the kidneys fail to reabsorb and thus spill glucose into urine, is about 180 mg/dl. The tight control that can be achieved today with blood glucose meters was much harder to accomplish.

This contributed to the diabetic retinopathy that I now have. Henry Dolger, MD, wrote the book I was given when diagnosed in 1960. He writes, "Clinitest, Clinistix, Galatest, or Tes-Tape are available. Since daily urine tests are needed in a great many cases, one of these is essential equipment. Clinistix only shows the presence or absence of sugar. The others also show the amount of sugar."[8]

Home Blood Glucose Monitoring

Home blood glucose monitoring came into use for the general public in about 1980. Before 1980, according to Dr. Joseph I. Goodman, a common way to have multiple readings for a twenty-four hour period was to have them done in the hospital. Dr. Goodman wrote in his 1978 book: "A blood glucose test can be processed within thirty minutes and even on the most modest schedule two hours should be adequate for any laboratory."[9] Now we can do it at home and have the result in five seconds, with only a small drop of blood.

My first glucose meter was an Ames that I purchased the summer of 1981. You had to be near a sink and have a large drop of blood to use it. The blood was placed on a strip, a button would be pushed on the meter, and a one-minute countdown would start. Once a minute elapsed, a high-pressure dose of water from a small bottle was applied to the strip, washing away what blood had not absorbed into the strip. The strip was then ready to be inserted into the meter for another one-minute countdown. Finally, after following these procedures, which took over two minutes, the result would be displayed. Do you see why the Way of Wisdom principle of good news and gratitude applies to what we have available for our use today? *"A cheerful look brings joy to the heart, and* **good news** *gives health to the bones"* (Proverbs 15:30). *"Like cold water to a weary soul is* **good news** *from a distant land"* (Proverbs 25:25).

Benefits of Routinely Checking Blood Glucose

The glucose meter is a blessing for which we can be very grateful! There are several benefits of regular glucose checking. Management of blood sugars can be much more effective. If the blood glucose is 200, for example, correction adjustments can be made for how much insulin to take for a meal—that is, if you use a rapid acting insulin like Novolog or Humalog. If you have Type 2 diabetes, knowing that the blood glucose is 200 would also help determine that a delay in eating is needed, or an avoidance of certain carbohydrates like rice or potatoes, which can rapidly drive up blood glucose levels. In fact, instead of eating at that time, a walk would be preferable first. All of these decisions can't be made when the blood glucose level is not known. By checking yourself, the guesswork can be taken out of management, giving you a sense of control. Another benefit is to feel better about the future, lowering the risk of complications by maintaining more normalized levels.

How to Overcome the Reluctance to Check Yourself

Why are some people so reluctant to use a meter? They may be looking at the glucose meter as a critic and not a friend. After all, when you purchase your strips, they are called *testing strips*, aren't they? Everyone remembers school and taking tests. We all got grades in school when we took a test.

In fact, there is story that illustrates the idea of looking at glucose strips as testing strips and the means people will go to get a passing grade. That's what happens when you take a test isn't it? You get a grade! In fact, there was research done on how accurate people were keeping their glucose records before the days when meters had a memory. It was discovered that many people were making up their numbers to take to the doctor, because unknown to them, they were using meters that actually did have a memory.

I like the story of a professor who gave a big test, the final of the semester to his students. He handed out all of the tests and went back to his desk to wait. Once the test was over, the students all handed the tests back. The professor noticed that one of the students had attached a hundred dollar bill to his test with a note saying "A dollar per point." During the next class, the professor handed the graded tests back to the students. The student who had handed his in with a hundred dollar bill received his back with sixty-four dollars attached. In other words, he got a thirty-six on his final exam. The last time I checked a thirty-six is an F, a failing grade.

Can you imagine applying a little blood to a strip, inserting it into the meter, and it comes back with a reading of 240 mg/dl? It is as though the meter is saying to you "You did it again. You flunked. That is a totally unacceptable number. You seem to always get Fs. You are such a loser." Is that what your meter is saying to you?

If you are always using the term *test strips* and are reluctant to use them, why not change the way you refer to them? Change *testing strips* to *checking* or *monitoring strips*. We've all heard the following saying: "Sticks and stones may break my bones, but words will never hurt me." We also know that words can indeed hurt us. The words in the following two paragraphs form pictures in our minds that are either uplifting or gloomy.

Read the following words very slowly: Unhappy, upset, tears, depressed, gloom, dark, sad, dismal, sullen, hopeless, bleak, sorrow, misery, somber, despair.

Now read these words very slowly: Joyful, joking, giggle, happy, laughter, glad, silly, cheerful, amusement, merriment, delightful, fun, jovial, jolly, hilarious.

Was there a difference in the pictures that were formed in your mind? Which paragraph encouraged you to get up and take on the challenges of the day? Words do affect us, don't they? The Way of Wisdom says, *"An anxious heart weighs a man down, but a kind word cheers him up"* (Proverbs 12:25). *"Pleasant words are like honey. They are sweet to the spirit and bring healing to the body"* (Proverbs 16:24).

Several years ago a football game was reported in the *Los Angeles Times*, at which more than a hundred people were hospitalized. A few people became ill at the game with symptoms of food poisoning. School officials ascertained that a soft drink dispensing machine under the stands might have been the culprit. They thought the soft drink mixture or tubing might have been contaminated. So school authorities had a public announcement made to not patronize the dispensing machine, because some people had become ill with food poisoning. When the announcement was made, the entire stadium became a sea of retching, fainting fans. Ambulances were called in from five hospitals, and more than a hundred people were hospitalized.

When it was found that the soft drink dispenser was entirely innocent, the illnesses vanished as quickly as they came. The critical agent in the whole incident was the language—food poisoning—both in causing the illnesses and in overcoming it.[10]

Is Your Glucose Meter a Critic, or Just an Informational Tool, Like the Fuel Gauge in Your Vehicle?

If you have problems with checking your blood glucose, it can be helpful to change the way you talk about it. Just changing the wording from *testing* to *monitoring* or *checking* can make a positive difference. Also, instead of thinking of it as a meter critic, think of it like you think of your vehicle fuel gauge. A fuel gauge for your vehicle provides you with information. I doubt you resent the fuel gauge and the information it provides about how much gas is left in your tank. Start checking your blood glucose, instead of testing it. After all, it is not really a test when you consider the hidden effects of stress on the levels, which we'll discuss in chapter eight. This is a small thing, but it can make a big difference! One woman says, "I can't stand to test myself. It hurts." Well, then she needs to *check* herself. It won't hurt as much, because she'll be looking at it in a more pleasant way. Think of checking a fuel gage for information, not of a test and meter critic. After all, God's wisdom says, *"Be careful what you think, because your thoughts run your life"* (Proverbs 4:23). *"Pleasant words are like honey. They are sweet to the spirit and bring healing to the body"* (Proverbs 16:24).

Where should your blood glucose be during the day? Here are some guidelines, with a comparison to normal numbers for those without diabetes.

Fasting and before breakfast: 70–130 mg/dl
Normal is less than 100 mg/dl

Before lunch, supper, and snacks: 70–130 mg/dl
Two hours after starting meals: 160 mg/dl or less
Normal is less than 140 mg/dl
Bedtime: 90–150 mg/dl
Normal is less than 120 mg/dl

What should your average be? 140 or less, which is an A1c of 6.5 percent or less, according to the American Association of Clinical Endocrinologists; or 7.0 percent or less is what it should be, according to the American Diabetes Association, which is 154 average. A normal A1c is considered 5.6 percent or less. If person's test result is a 5.7 to 6.4 percent that person is considered to have prediabetes and is at high risk for developing diabetes.[11] The following formula can be used to determine what an average blood sugar is based upon the A1c result:

$(A1c \times 28.7) - 46.7$ = average blood sugar

What is the A1c?

A1c hemoglobin is a protein that carries oxygen around the body. It is packaged within the red blood cell, which lives for about ninety days. Glucose in the blood attaches or sticks to the hemoglobin. In everyone without diabetes or prediabetes 4 to 5.6 percent is covered with glucose. Of course, the higher your blood glucose average is, the greater the percentage number will be. About half of the percentage value reflects the last thirty days' blood glucose levels.[12]

How many times a day should you check?

Check your blood glucose as many times as it takes per day to get the above averages. Use the pair method. The pair method is checking your blood glucose before a meal like lunch and then checking it two hours after you began to eat. Do this for three days in a row, logging what you ate and what exercise you did. You will then be able to see the effects certain kinds of food have on your blood sugar levels. You can do the same thing for breakfast and supper. For information on what to do if you experience a low blood sugar of 70 mg/dl or less, read chapter 6. If you need additional strips at a low cost of about 18 cents apiece, go to www.americandiabeteswholesale.com.

From No Medications to an Assortment of Medications

Back in 1958, Dr. Henry Dolger wrote, "Certainly the immediate impact of Orinase on the treatment of diabetes has been extraordinary. In June, 1957, when the drug was first released by the FDA, about 20,000 patients had used it....This goes far beyond the obvious fact that it is easier to swallow Orinase tablets than to plunge a hypodermic needle into one's skin every day."[13]

Today there are an assortment of medications that have different functions. Some stimulate the pancreas to produce and release more insulin (for people with Type 2). The first-generation drug was Orinase, but the current medications are Glipizide, Glimeperide, and Glyburide. Other medications help cells to be sensitive to insulin. Metformin decreases the liver's production of glucose, resulting in better fasting glucose levels in the morning.[14] Other newer medications relate to hormones called *incretins*. Januvia and Onglyza are two of these medications.

The most significant incretin hormone for diabetes management is called *glucagon-like peptide-1*

(GLP-1). Basically, it is a messenger that is activated by incoming nutrients. It then stimulates the beta cells in the islets of Langerhans to produce insulin while food is being eaten. It comes from the small intestine. It also suppresses the secretion of a hormone called *gluca-gon*, which releases stored glucose in the liver. GLP-1 also suppresses appetite. The amount of secretion of GLP-1 is decreased in people with Type 2 diabetes. As the amount is already reduced and is rapidly inactivated by an enzyme called DPP-4, people with Type 2 diabetes end up with elevated blood glucose levels after eating. Inhibitors to the DPP-4 enzyme, like Januvia and Onglyza, have now been developed, thus giving the GLP-1 more time to stimulate the beta cells in the pancreas to keep producing insulin while one eats.[15]

Now that we've examined some of the medications that have been developed over the last fifty years, we can realize what good news we have for today! It would be easy to complain about the cost as well as the hassle of remembering to take the medication(s) at the right time and the right amount. Now that we've looked back at the past experiences of others who were trying to cope with diabetes, however, was it a shock to learn how few resources were available? What do we do with this information? How can we apply wisdom's instruction to this? That is what we will begin to examine in the next chapter.

"Where there is no revelation, people cast off restraint; but blessed are those who heed wisdom's instruction" (Proverbs 29:18).

---

1. Michael Bliss, *The Discovery of Insulin* (Chicago: The University of Chicago Press, 1982), 161, 164.
2. Bliss, 72, 78.

3. Richard Beaser, MD, ed., *Joslin Diabetes Deskbook: A Guide for Primary Care Providers* (Boston: Joslin Diabetes Center, 2010), 4, 5.

4. Beaser, 5.

5. Bliss, 150–51

6. Richard Jackson, MD, and Amy Tenderich, *Know Your Numbers, Outlive Your Diabetes: Five Essential Health Factors You Can Master to Enjoy a Long and Healthy Life* (New York: Marlowe & Company, 2007), 43–44.

7. William H. Polonsky, *Diabetes Burnout: What to Do When You Can't Take It Anymore* (Alexandria, Virginia: American Diabetes Association, 1999), 97.

8. Henry Dolger, MD, and Bernard Seeman, *How to Live with Diabetes* (New York: Pyramid Books, Inc., 1958), 85.

9. Joseph I. Goodman, MD, *Diabetes without Fear* (New York: Avon Books, 1978), 42.

10. Norman Cousins, *Head First: The Biology of Hope* (New York: E. P. Dutton, 1989), 82.

11. http://www.diabetes.org/diabetes-basics/diagnosis/ (Accessed May 21, 2013).

12. Jackson and Tenderich, 20.

13. Dolger and Seeman, 104–05, 109.

14. Jackson and Tenderich, 43–44.

15. Beaser, 212, 214.

Chapter 3

Placing the Wisdom Principle of Gratitude at the Center of Motivation

"Trust in the LORD with all your heart and lean not on your own understanding; in all your ways acknowledge him, and he will make your paths straight" (Proverbs 3:5–6). *Trust* is the first word he says in this passage. Trust is a concept that includes the idea of safety, confidence, and security. In other words, one can get a sense of security and safety by following God's wisdom. A good analogy of this is the safety belts that construction workers wear while working on water towers or high-rise buildings. People have made fatal mistakes by not staying hooked to their safety gear.

We, too, can stay safe by keeping our trust in God. We are to trust, putting our confidence in God's ways. When we unhook our belt of trust, it can lead to discouragement, despair, and lack of discipline. We can fall into the pleasure trap of just being a couch potato, eating whatever we desire, thinking we are exempt from any problems that could arise from elevated blood sugar levels. We can unhook that belt of trust by feeling sorry for ourselves and complaining.

You may have heard the story of the man who went to a monastery in the Himalayan mountains. This was a place where words were few. Each resident was only allowed to speak two words every seven years when they were brought before their superior. After his first seven years, his superior asked him, "What are your words?" He said, "Bed's hard!" Then after fourteen years, the same thing happened, except this time he said, "Food's bad!" Finally, after being there for twenty-one years, he said, "I quit!" To that, his superior replied, "I'm not surprised. The only thing you've done since you got here is complain." We do not have to be like that man, do we?

Instead, what we can do is trust in God and always be looking for what is good. *"He who seeks good finds goodwill, but evil comes to him who searches for it"* (Proverbs 11:27). When we look for the positive, we will find it. *"A cheerful look brings joy to your heart. And good news gives health to your body"* (Proverbs 15:30).

An important part of the good news is that we can keep learning. Things don't have to stay the way they are today. Life and health can improve. When we trust in God's way, his way of wisdom, our ways will be kept straight. When it comes to learning, the way of wisdom states: *"The mind of a person with understanding gets knowledge; the wise person listens to learn more"* (Proverbs 18:15). *"Anyone who gets wisdom loves himself. Anyone who values understanding succeeds"* (Proverbs 19:8).

The idea of continuing to learn is just as relevant today as it was in 1923. Dr. Elliott Joslin, who was a leading specialist in the care of people with diabetes, and for whom the Joslin Diabetes Center in Boston is named, stated in his *Diabetic Manual for Doctor and Patient*, "The patient is his own nurse, doctor's assistant and chemist. To acquire the requisite knowledge for this triple vocation requires diligent study, but the prize often is worthwhile for it is nothing less than life itself."[1] We need to have the attitude to learn as much as we can, so we don't fall into fatal attitude mistakes. When I said to one church leader that I have diabetes, he said, "That's no big deal. Almost everyone has diabetes." That man's fatal attitude mistake was underrating diabetes, not realizing how serious its effects can be on health.

I've heard people say, "I just have a touch of diabetes" or "I'm just borderline." One person said, "My fasting blood sugar was only 110, so I'm ok." However, according to the Centers for Disease Control a level like that would indicate prediabetes rather than being ok! After an eight hour fast, people who have glucose levels of 100 to 125 mg/dL are considered to have impaired fasting glucose (IFG). Another test is the oral glucose tolerance test. It is also administered after an eight hour fast, but people first drink a liquid which contains about 75 grams of glucose. If the result is 140 to 199 mg/dL they have impaired glucose tolerance. Both of these results indicate prediabetes and 15% to 30% of those with this condition, without any lifestyle changes, will have Type 2 Diabetes within five years.[2]

Dr. John R. Williams in Rochester, New York, just across Lake Ontario from Toronto, was the first American doctor given insulin to use. His first patient, and the first American to receive insulin, was James D. Havens. He was diagnosed at the age of about fifteen. When he received his first dose of insulin he was a skeletal twenty-two-year-old. He had lived for more than seven years on Dr. Frederick Allen's "under-nutrition" therapy or starvation diet. For periods of time, he would eat only two hundred calories a day to keep his blood sugar from spilling over into his urine. (And we think it's difficult to *cut back* two hundred calories a day.)

By the spring of 1922, he weighed seventy-three-and-a-half pounds, was too weak to sit up in bed, and cried in pain most of the time. On May 21, 1922, when it appeared that James had only a few days to live, he became the first American to receive insulin. He lived another thirty-eight years and died, not of complications from diabetes, but from colon cancer. James wrote to Dr. Banting, the discoverer of insulin: "A week ago last Thursday....Marked an historical event as I then tasted my first egg and toast. Egg on toast is my idea of the only food necessary in heaven."[3] From the example of James, two wisdom principles can be learned: diligence and gratitude. We'll look at gratitude now and diligence in chapter 12.

Trusting in the Lord with Gratitude

"A cheerful look brings joy to your heart. And good news gives health to your body" (Proverbs 15:30). We can be thankful today that we don't have to endure what James Havens had to face. His comment after receiving insulin was a comment of gratitude! When I realize we have so many new resources available today like glucose meters, new types of insulin, insulin pumps and pens, and assortment of medications, and other ways to prevent or cope with complications that weren't available more than fifty years ago, I am overwhelmed

with gratitude! I believe this gratitude perspective can help anyone face the challenge to outsmart diabetes when used on a daily basis.

Some People Count Their Blessings While Others Think Their Blessings Don't Count

This principle of gratitude has been lost in recent published books and articles for diabetes management. Way back in 1942, however, Dr. Elliott Joslin advocated to his patients to "be cheerful and also be thankful that his disease is not of a hopeless character, but a disease which his brains will help him conquer."[4] One of his patients, John Hansen, was diagnosed with diabetes in 1940 at the age of fifteen. In 1959, he expressed his attitude by writing, "I have been grateful for every day of life I have had since first becoming diabetic. I've always regarded each day as a sort of bonus."[5] As I've mentioned, we have so many more ways to outsmart diabetes than John had back in 1959, but we still need the motivation to do so. Gratitude, when properly applied, will provide the motivation!

Students at Oxford heard that Rudyard Kipling (author of *The Jungle Book* and *The Man Who Would Be King*) was making about fifty cents for every word he wrote, which equals about ten dollars per word today. This was about 1900. They cabled a message to him with fifty cents, asking him for one of his very best words. He sent back "THANKS!" *Thanks* is one of our very best words, worth a lot to the person who hears it and to the person who lives it. Why, then, isn't it used more and heard more? It seems that it has never been used much. After Jesus healed the ten lepers, only one came back and said thanks. Paul wrote, *"and be thankful"* (Colossians 3:15).

When It Gets Dark Enough, You Can See the Stars

The late Dr. Lee Salk, formerly of Cornell University Medical College, wrote about his mother's experiences as a girl growing up in Russia. She was driven from her home by the Cossacks. They burned her village, and she had to flee for her life, hiding in hay wagons and ditches. She eventually got on a crowded ship and made it to America. Dr. Salk writes, "Even after my mother married and her sons were born...it was a struggle to keep food on the table....But my mother urged us to think about what we had, not what we didn't have. She taught us that in hardship you develop a capacity to appreciate the beauty that exists in the simplest elements of life. The attitude that she so fiercely conveyed to us was this: 'When it gets dark enough, you can see the stars.'"[6]

When a person is diagnosed with diabetes or a complication from diabetes, it may seem dark, but let's remember that the stars are always there. We just don't notice them in the daytime of life, when everything seems to be going well. We take them for granted, just like so many other good things or blessings in our lives. We do not always focus on the things we already have, the things for which we can be thankful. Instead, we often are looking for things we don't have. Let's focus on all that is available to help us outsmart diabetes, use what is available, and be thankful! Now, along with God's wisdom, scientific research also indicates how beneficial being grateful can be for health and wellness. Let's trust in God by using his wisdom, because the way of wisdom states that *good news gives health to your body* (Proverbs 15:30). The natural response to good news is not to complain and feel deprived, but rather to be thankful and excited!

Count Your Blessings and You Will Show a Profit. Have the Attitude of Gratitude. Look on the Brighter Side of Life—The Good News.

"A cheerful heart makes you healthy. But a broken spirit dries you up" (Proverbs 17:22). *"Hearing good news from a land far away is like drinking cold water when you are tired"* (Proverbs 25:25).

Let's now look at the scientific research on gratitude and then a practical way to make gratitude a part of our lifestyle for managing any chronic illness.

1. Donald M. Barnett, MD, *Elliott P. Joslin, MD: A Centennial Portrait* (Boston: Joslin Diabetes Center, 1998), 35.

2. Centers for Disease Control (2012, October 5). Prediabetes Facts. http://www.cdc.gov/diabetes/prevention/factsheet.htm (Accessed June 17, 2013)

3. Thea Cooper and Arthur Ainsberg, *Breakthrough: Elizabeth Hughes, the Discovery of Insulin, and the Making of a Medical Miracle* (New York: St. Martin's Press, 2010), 168–69.

4. Chris Feudtner, MD, *Bittersweet: Diabetes, Insulin, and the Transformation of Illness* (Chapel Hill: The University of North Carolina Press, 2003), 115.

5. Feudtner, 191.

6. Alan Loy McGinnis, *The Power of Optimism* (San Francisco: Harper & Row Publishers, 1990), 74.

Chapter 4

Counting Blessings: Some People Count Their Blessings While Others Discount Theirs— Gratitude Research

---
It is a Matter of Perspective

I read about a feisty ninety-one-year-old grandmother, living alone, who had to have complete hip replacement surgery. Of course, after the surgery she was housebound. Her family, who didn't live nearby, was very concerned about her welfare. The family wanted her to participate in a local "Meals on Wheels" program, so that warm meals could be brought to her.

The grandmother was a very independent lady and did not like the idea of being considered helpless, so tact had to be used to get her to participate. A volunteer phoned her and cheerfully explained the Meals on Wheels program and how it really relies on volunteers to help the elderly and the ill. The volunteer asked, "Would you be interested in it?" There was a contemplative pause. "Well, sure," the grandmother said. "If you can't find anyone else to get food to the old people, I guess I can." I like that woman's perspective, don't you? She didn't think of herself as a victim, but as a helper! Life is a matter of perspective, isn't it?

I heard about a man celebrating his hundredth birthday. A local television reporter went to interview him. The reporter asked, "Are you able to get out and walk much?" He replied with a radiant grin, "Well, I certainly walk better today than I could a hundred years ago." I like that man's perspective, too! He automatically and humorously thought of some advantages he has today! Life is really influenced by our perspective, isn't it? How can we use perspective to our advantage when it comes to the challenges we face in our own lives? What difference would it make to be looking at life through the lens or perspective of gratitude? It has been said that...

"Appreciation is like looking through a wide-angle lens
that lets you see the entire forest, not just the one tree
limb you walked up on."

If we constantly remind ourselves of our blessings, it makes it harder to take them for granted. If we don't take them for granted, and instead have the perspective of gratitude for them, will that make any difference in our overall health and well-being? A ten-week research study with hundreds of participants was done by professor Robert Emmons, PhD, of University of California at Davis to demonstrate what effects gratitude might have on health and well-being. They were randomly divided into three groups. One group was a gratitude condition group, and the members were to list five things for which they could be thankful that had affected their lives from the previous week. Another group was the hassle group, and those people were to list five burdens that affected their lives the previous week. The third group was the neutral group, and its members were to list five things, either positive or negative, that had affected their lives the previous week.

The results were then analyzed with several tests. The final analysis was that the people in the gratitude group felt better about their lives, were more optimistic, and exercised more than those in the other groups. The results were even better when gratitude was practiced on a daily basis, looking at a variety of blessings.[1]

Several other studies have been conducted, with similar results. For example, another ten-week study was done by the Department of Physical Medicine and Rehabilitation at the University of Cal-Davis, involving people with post-polio syndrome. The results of the gratitude group was that the people felt better about themselves, felt more optimistic about the coming week, and felt more connected with others than the other groups. Another significant finding was that they went to sleep quicker, spent more time sleeping, and felt more refreshed in the morning.[2] The idea is that if you want to sleep more soundly, count your blessings, not sheep.

Other research studies also demonstrate how beneficial appreciation and gratitude can be to a person's well-being. By keeping a daily gratitude journal, individuals, including the chronically ill, find themselves feeling generally better, more optimistic, and more connected to others. Seventy-four transplant recipients (of either heart, liver, lung, kidney, or pancreas) who expressed gratitude felt physically better than those who didn't.[3]

Is a grateful heart a healthy heart? In the context of receiving a new heart, what good is feeling grateful? A University of Pittsburgh study of 119 heart transplant patients found that being appreciative and thankful positively related to perceived feelings of physical and mental health one year later. Thankfulness was also predictive of better compliance with a meal plan and medications.[4]

Another research study related to the effects of stress was also done. After a month of a daily, fifteen-minute practice of appreciation, a research group had an increase in a hormone called dehydroepiandros-terone (which reflects physiological relaxation) and a reduction in cortisol. Cortisol and stress will be discussed in chapter 8.

How can this research help with the motivation needed to manage diabetes or other chronic diseases? If you want to be more optimistic about the coming week, feel more connected with others, sleep better, have better compliance with a meal plan and medications, exercise more, and reduce levels of the stress hormone cortisol, then practice gratitude.

The apostle Paul also wrote that gratitude and not giving up go together like a hand in a glove. To the church at Colossae he wrote, *"May you be made strong with all the strength that comes from his glorious power, and may you be prepared to **endure every-thing** with patience, **while joyfully giving thanks** to the Father"* (Colossians 1:11–12). In the next chapter, we'll examine a useful way to practice gratitude and make it an integral part of managing diabetes! Remember, the way of wisdom teaches us to be grateful by focusing on good news, which results in better health! Notice how wisdom itself is good news, because using it can result in a healthier, longer life; better decision making; and a more pleasant, peaceful lifestyle.

Gratitude for Wisdom's Rewards: A Healthier, Longer, More Wholesome Life

"Lay hold of my words with all your heart; keep my commands and you will live. Get wisdom, get understanding; do not forget my words or swerve from them. Do not forsake wisdom, and she will protect you; love her, and she will watch over you. Wisdom is supreme; therefore get wisdom. Though it cost all you have, get understanding. Esteem her, and she will exalt you; embrace her, and she will honor you. She will set a garland of grace on your head and present you with a crown of splendor. Listen, my son, accept what I say, and the years of your life will be many. I guide you in the way of wisdom and lead you along straight paths. When you walk, your steps will not be hampered; when you run, you will not stumble. Hold on to instruction, do not let it go; guard it well, for it is your life" (Proverbs 4:4–13).

Gratitude for Wisdom's Advantages: Discernment, Understanding (Better Decision Making)

"Then you will understand respect for the Lord, and you will find that you know God. Only the Lord gives wisdom; he gives knowledge and understanding. He stores up wisdom for those who are honest. Like a shield he protects the innocent. He makes sure that justice is done, and he protects those who are loyal to him. Then you will understand what is honest and fair and what is the good and right thing to do. Wisdom will come into your mind, and knowledge will be pleasing to you. Good sense will protect you; understanding will guard you" (Proverbs 2:5–11).

Gratitude for the Value of Wisdom, Which Brings a Pleasant, Peaceful Lifestyle

---

"Blessed is the one who finds wisdom. Blessed is the one who gains understanding. Wisdom pays better than silver does. She earns more than gold does. She is worth more than rubies. Nothing you want can compare with her. Long life is in her right hand. In her left hand are riches and honor. Her ways are pleasant ways. All her paths lead to peace. She is a tree of life to those who hold her close. Those who hold on to her will be blessed" (Proverbs 3:13–18).

The Guidelines of Wisdom for Health and Wellness

"My son, do not forget my teaching. Keep my commands in your heart. They will help you live for many years. They will bring you success....Don't be wise in your own eyes. Have respect for the LORD and avoid evil. That will bring health to your body. It will make your bones strong" (Proverbs 3:1–2, 7–8).

"A tranquil heart makes for a healthy body, but jealousy is [like] bone cancer" (Proverbs 14:30). "A cheerful look brings joy to your heart. And good news gives health to your body" (Proverbs 15:30). "Pleasant words are like honey. They are sweet to the spirit and bring healing to the body" (Proverbs 16:24).

How can wisdom be defined? Wisdom was used to describe a skill that a person had in a given area of life (compare 1 Kings 7:14). Notice the qualities with which it is associated in the following passage: *"I, wisdom, dwell together with prudence; I possess knowledge and discretion. To fear the LORD is to hate evil; I hate pride and arrogance, evil behavior and perverse speech. Counsel and sound judgment are mine; I have understanding and power"* (Proverbs 8:12-14). Wisdom goes hand in glove with prudence, discretion, sound judgment and understanding. All of these qualities empower a person to live effectively. **Therefore, wisdom can be defined as having the skill for living.**

A person is not born with wisdom, but it is a quality or skill that is learned (Read Proverbs 2:1-6, 18:15). Those who learn wisdom use it in their own lives as well as teach others to be wise. You may have heard the saying "Give a man a fish and you feed him for a day; teach a man how to fish and you feed him for a lifetime." Here is how the concept is put in Proverbs: *"A good person gives life to others; the wise person teaches others how to live"* (Proverbs 11:30). Wisdom is more valuable than anything we may desire because it will affect every area of our lives, including our health (Proverbs 3:15, 4:22). The following is an example of how valuable wisdom was for a person who was facing every privation.

At the end of World War II the condition of prisoners in concentration camps was horrific. American soldiers were assigned to give medical help to the newly liberated prisoners. George Ritchie was one of the soldiers assigned to a team to do this. He described it as the most shattering experience he had yet had, seeing "the effects of slow starvation, to walk through those barracks where thousands of men had died a little bit at a time over a period of years." The paperwork alone was staggering in trying to relocate these people whose families and even hometowns had disappeared. His team came across one of the prisoners who could help. It was obvious that he hadn't been there long: his posture was erect, his eyes bright, his energy unending. Since he was fluent in English, French, German and Russian, as well as Polish, he became a kind of unofficial camp translator. His compassion for his fellow-prisoners glowed on his face, and it was to this glow that Ritchie would turn when his own spirits were low.

Ritchie was astonished when this man's papers came before him for processing. He had been there since 1939! Ritchie says, "For six years he had lived on the same starvation diet, slept in the same airless and disease-ridden barracks as everyone else, but without the least physical or mental deterioration." "It's not easy for some of them to forgive," Ritchie commented to him one day as they sat over mugs of tea in the processing center. He said, "So many of them have lost members of their families." Hatred among them ran high toward the Germans. Then for the first time he spoke of himself, his wife, two daughters and three little boys. He told how he and his family lived in the Jewish section of Warsaw and how when the Germans came they lined up everyone, including his family. He begged to die with his family, but because he spoke German they put him in a work group.

He said, "I had to decide right then whether to let myself hate the soldiers who had done this." His decision was easy though because in his practice as a lawyer he had already seen what hate could do to people's lives. Hate had just killed his family. He said, "I decided then that I would spend the rest of my life— whether it was a few days or many years—loving every person I came in contact with."[5]

What kept this man thriving while being confronted with every privation? Love is what kept him well! Love is an attribute of God's wisdom. The following are two proverbs of God's wisdom concerning love: *"Hatred stirs up dissension, but love covers over all wrongs"* (Proverbs 10:12). *"He who covers over an offense promotes love, but whoever repeats the matter separates close friends"* (Proverbs 17:9). By practicing the teachings of those two proverbs concerning love this man was empowered to endure. If he could live through such horrible circumstances, surely we can meet the challenges we may face daily with diabetes! And we can, if we do so with God's wisdom! That's why wisdom is included in this chapter on gratitude because it is something for which we can be thankful and is far more valuable than anything else we might desire. *"Choose my instruction instead of silver, knowledge rather than choice gold, for wisdom is more precious than rubies, and nothing you desire can compare with her"* (Proverbs 8:10-11).

---

1. Robert A. Emmons, *Thanks: How Practicing Gratitude Can Make You Happier* (New York: Houghton Mifflin Company, 2007), 27. Emmons, 32–33.

2. Stephen Post, *Why Good Things Happen to Good People: The Exciting New Research That Proves the Link Between Doing Good and Living a Longer, Healthier, Happier Life* (New York: Broadway Books, 2007), 28, 30.

3. Emmons, 66.

4. Emmons, 73.

5. George G. Ritchie, and Elizabeth Sherrill, *Return from Tomorrow* (Grand Rapids, MI: Baker Publishing Group, 1978, 2007), 131.

Chapter 5

Practicing Gratitude on a Daily Basis to Stay Motivated

God's wisdom instructs us to focus on the good, on our blessings. *"He who seeks good finds goodwill, but evil comes to him who searches for it"* (Proverbs 11:27). *"Like cold water to a weary soul is good news from a distant land"* (Proverbs 25:25). I like to hear good news, don't you? And it doesn't have to be from a distant land. Suppose you have a new house, and you are cleaning one of the closets and find this note: "Because of my concern that some of my greedy, ungrateful children would squander my money once I am gone, I decided to bury $1,500,000 in the backyard near the giant oak tree. The money is located in a metal box approximately three feet to the left of the tree and nine inches beneath the surface. If you find it, it's yours." It's signed by the previous owner of the house.

How would you respond? Would you keep cleaning? Would you be thinking, "Someday it might be nice to dig around in the backyard and see if I can find that box?" Or would you think "Since I don't know for sure whether the letter and its author are trustworthy, I'll just disregard the note?" NO! I suspect you would get a shovel and start digging! Did you know that God is offering you something far more valuable than one-and-a-half million dollars? It's called *wisdom*. Let's not put off practicing it today! If you don't have any good news from a distant land, like the proverb says, then what are you to do? Look in your own backyard.

It's Been Said, "If You Can't See the Bright Side, Then Polish the Dull Side."

If the grass looks greener on the other side of the fence, then look more thoroughly on your own side. It's been said that if you can't see the bright side, polish the dull side. We have good news happening in our lives every day! That is why the apostle Paul said, *"Give thanks in all circumstances, for this is God's will for you in Christ Jesus"* (1 Thessalonians 5:18). He didn't say to be thankful *for* all circumstances, but *in* those circumstances search out things for which you can be thankful.

What is a practical way to use this wisdom principle of gratitude? Consider the following example that at one time was listed on cnn.com: You've got a pounding headache, your morning newspaper is soggy, and your shoelace just broke. When you stop to buy a cup of coffee, the clerk greets you with: "Good morning! How are you doing today?" You say, "My head hurts, and I'm irritated as can be. Just give me my coffee." (I'm honest.) What about the following answer: You say,

"I'm blessed and fine. How are you?" (Yep, I'd lie.) Then the article commented, "Social lies, or white lies, are so common, most people wouldn't even call them lies. The intent is not to deceive, but to respect the other person's sensitivity."

"Feel Bad Page" or "Feel Good Page"

Do you agree with that conclusion? I don't agree, because there is a concept that many people have never even considered. It is the concept of a "Feel Bad Page" and a "Feel Good Page." It's the same concept as in the saying, "When it gets dark enough, you can see the stars." The stars are always there, just like there is always a "Feel Bad Page" and a "Feel Good Page" happening in each person's life. It is simply a matter of deciding from which page a person chooses to read!

It's easy to complain about the bad things that are happening in one's life, but it seems to take more effort to think about the good things. When we consider all the things we have available today to help manage diabetes, compared to how it's been in the past, we can put those things on a "Feel Good Page" and be thankful. Many medications that we've mentioned, like Januvia and Metformin; new insights into nutrition and movement; and new tools like insulin pens, insulin pumps, and glucose meters can all be listed on the "Feel Good Page." The way of wisdom teaches us to focus on that page!

Keeping Good Records

If you were instructed to keep good records of your blood sugar readings, the amount of food you eat each day, and the number of steps you take each day, would you say "You've got to be kidding"? Or "I've never done such a silly thing"? The way of wisdom, however, states the concept with this principle: *"Be sure you know the condition of your flocks"* (Proverbs 27:23). Most of us do not have flocks, but each of us does have a body, and we need to keep track of the condition of our blood glucose levels, blood pressure, cholesterol, micro albumin (kidney function), and so on. In other words, we need to keep a daily personal health inventory. One way to do this is to keep a food diary along with records of blood glucose readings.

In the *Journal of the American Dietetic Association*, an article titled "Food Records: A Predictor and Modifier of Weight Change in a Long-Term Weight Loss Program" concluded: "Those who most accurately recorded their food consumption lost the most weight."[1] Keeping records is one of the most important things we can do. What important feature is usually missing from a food/ glucose record-keeping diary? A gratitude diary!

I've got what I call my "Tasty Eating Food Diary and Outsmarting Diabetes Record Booklet." On each page I have five lines for listing good things. It is help-ful to keep a list of gifts or blessings that varies, so that the daily list doesn't become redundant, having the same things every day. We don't even have to do this every day to benefit from this practice, as the research indicates. In the research that was examined in the last chapter, Dr. Emmons had three research groups, which were to focus on listing either blessings from the previ-ous week, or problems, or a combination of both. When he came to the group where the members were to just list hassles or problems, he wrote, "We have never found a research participant who has had any difficulty in understanding what we were asking for or coming up with a list of problems."[2] What about blessings, though? What kinds of things can we list?

From the research of Dr. Emmons, when the gratitude group listed their blessings, they fell into two major categories: focusing on self or others. Some listed things like "my health, strength"; "my mind and thinking rationally"; "my strong will and desire"; or "receiving money from my Grandma." Their blessings tended to be self-directed or centered. With that focus, it was harder for them to list blessings. In contrast, the other category of people tended to have more blessings focused on others, like "my family, especially my child to come"; "the support I receive from those around me"; "God's help through difficult times"; "my caring husband"; "having food on the table." With that kind of focus, it was much easier for that group's members to list their blessings.[3]

Based upon that research, it would be more beneficial to include little things that others do to enrich our lives when we make our list. When we keep our focus on the good things, listing them on our "Feel Good Page," they will all contribute to maintaining a positive attitude. A positive attitude is what we all need to have to keep doing the things we need to do on a daily basis. *"A man's spirit sustains him in sickness, but a crushed spirit who can bear?"* (Proverbs 18:14).

Gifts

Another helpful way to think of good things or blessings is to view them as gifts. Again, according to recent research, to be more grateful, view your blessings as gifts. But, of course, God in his wisdom has been teaching this for thousands of years. *"She* (that is, God's wisdom) *will set a garland of **grace** on your head and* present *you with a crown of splendor"* (Proverbs 4:9). To Timothy, the apostle Paul wrote, *"I am **thankful** to Christ Jesus our Lord. He has given me strength. I **thank** him that he considered me faithful. And I **thank** him for appointing me to serve him. I used to speak evil things against Jesus. I tried to hurt his followers. I really pushed them around. But God showed me mercy anyway. I did those things without knowing any better. I wasn't a believer. Our Lord poured out more and more of his **grace*** (or gift) *on me"* (1 Timothy 1:12–14).

Yet another study was done at Cal-Davis University by Dr. Emmons on perceiving good things as gifts. The following instructions were given to participants: "Focus for a moment on benefits or 'gifts' that you have received in your life. These gifts could be every-day pleasures, people in your life, personal strengths or talents, moments of natural beauty or gestures of kind-ness from others. We might not normally think about these things as gifts, but that is how we want you to think about them. Take a moment to really savor or rel-ish these 'gifts,' think about their value, and then write them down in the spaces below."[4]

Half of the gifts listed related to "interpersonal" or "spiritual" categories. When these categories were viewed not as just good things, but as gifts, the par-ticipants were able to come up with 20 percent more things to list. According to the research, these are the categories of blessings that relate to better health and well-being. Research also indicated that the more a receiver valued the gift, the greater he or she experi-enced gratitude. So instead of just thinking of oral med-ications, glucose meters and checking strips, insulin, knowledge of the glycemic index—in other words, the resources that were not even available years ago for people to use—as merely *good things,* think of them as gifts. And let's not forget to cherish the supportive people in our lives as gifts as well!

"Interpersonal" Or "Spiritual" Categories Illustration

Fred Craddock tells the story of a missionary family in China who was forced to leave the country sometime after the communists took over. One day a band of soldiers knocked on the door and told this missionary, his wife, and children that they had two hours to pack up before these troops would escort them to the train station. They would be permitted to take with them only two hundred pounds of stuff.

Thus began two hours of family wrangling and bickering: what should they take? What about this vase? It's a family heirloom, so we've got to take the vase. Well, maybe so, but this typewriter is brand new and we're not about to leave that behind. What about some books? We've got to take a few of them along. On and on it went, putting stuff on the bathroom scale and taking it off until finally they had a pile of possessions that totaled two hundred pounds on the dot.

At the appointed hour, the soldiers returned. "Are you ready?" they asked this missionary family. "Yes." "Did you weigh your stuff?" "Yes, we did." "Do you have just two hundred pounds?" "Yes, we only have two hundred pounds exactly." "Did you weigh the kids?" "Um, no; weigh the kids!"

In an instant the vase, the typewriter, and the books all became trash. Trash! None of it meant anything compared to the surpassing value of the children. That illustration really demonstrates the value most people place on "interpersonal" relationships and how they can be perceived as gifts. Of course, the result is a greater feeling of gratitude. According to the research, gratitude for this category of blessings results in better health and wellness. Let's focus on interactions with and encouragement from others as gifts that we can list in our gratitude journals.

Remember a Time...

Another way to think of good things as gifts is to remember a time when you felt grateful for what someone did for you that made a profound difference in your life. What would have happened if someone had not stepped forward and helped you?

The following is a personal example that directly relates to gifts and diabetes management. When my wife and I and our two little boys had moved to the Kansas City area in 1986, one afternoon I experienced a traumatic event—a hemorrhage in my left eye. We were walking around a lake at Watkins Mill State Park, pulling a little red wagon with our two little boys in it. I began to notice a small dot in my left eye, which continued to grow. I was experiencing a hemorrhage into the vitreous of my eye. I didn't know any doctors in the area, and it was a Saturday, but I was able to contact an ophthalmologist, who told me there was no way to stop it while it was happening. I went to his office on Monday. He looked at my eye and said I would have to wait for some of the blood to be absorbed by the body before laser treatment could be used on the retina. He told me the only thing I could do now was pray. I said I was already doing that.

Fortunately, a new friend in our church informed me of a specialist—an endocrinologist—in Kansas City, Dr. Richard Hellman. I saw him almost immediately, and he then referred me to an ophthalmologist, Dr. Matthew

Ziemianski. The news of the hemorrhage was distressing enough, but add to that the discovery that my health insurance company had just gone bankrupt too...it made the situation overwhelmingly stressful! While sitting in the waiting room with my wife and two little boys, the doctor's nurse overheard a conversation I was having with another patient about my situation. She then informed the doctor.

So when I went into the doctor's office, he made a statement that I still get emotional about to this day, almost twenty-seven years later. He said his nurse had told him of my situation. Then he told me that he would do laser treatment on my eyes without charge! I remember his words as if they were spoken yesterday: "Those boys need a father who can see." He used the pan-retinal laser photocoagulation treatment in both eyes, which was developed by Dr. Lloyd M. Aiello of the Joslin Diabetes Center, and thus saved my vision (now 20/20 and 20/25). Those words and what he did were truly gifts to me. I experienced the way of wisdom's principle of gratitude in a profound way from that experience. Remember, the principle is found in Proverbs 15:30: *"Good news gives health to your body."* To get started, go to your own memories and think of a time when someone did something significant for you. Did you really deserve it? Was it expected? Then think of it as a gift! Choose to think of good news and good things as gifts for which you can be abundantly grateful. It will make a positive difference in your health and your life!

One Appreciative Day at a Time

It's easy to be caught up looking at the past with the wrong perspective, only thinking about things that should have been done or shouldn't have been done. We can begin to fall into the "If only" trap. If only I had been using my time more wisely, taking the time to exercise more, and so on. This is a gloomy approach that only leads to a downward pull of discouragement. It's like a man who is being chased by a tiger (the depressing things from the past); he runs until he comes to a sheer cliff. As the tiger bears down on him, he grabs a rope dangling over the cliff and climbs down out of the tiger's reach. He looks and sees the tiger growling at him. Then he looks down and sees a deadly drop to the rocky floor about five hundred feet below. Then he looks up and sees two mice beginning to chew on the rope. What should he do?

The tiger is above, the rocks are below, the rope is about to break! Just then he spots a bright red, ripe strawberry, growing out of the side of the cliff. He stretches out his hand, plucks the strawberry, and pops it into his mouth. The juices are so sweet that, as he eats, he can't contain himself and says, "Delicious—that's the best strawberry I've ever tasted."

Had the man been preoccupied with the tiger (the *depressing past*) or preoccupied with the rocks below (the *future*), he would never have enjoyed the strawberry, which we call the *precious present*! Let's live in the precious present while managing diabetes, doing the best we can each day by looking at all the good things we have, like the strawberry this man had. We can also bring blessings or gifts from the past to also help enjoy the precious present. As Thomas Carlyle wrote, "Our main business is not to see what lies dimly at a distance, but to do what lies clearly at hand." If we look at things from the past with the attitude of gratitude, those things at a distance will be bright, not dim!

Let's live in day-tight compartments, making each day a "Feel Good Page" day, doing as the psalmist instructed: *"This is the day the LORD has made. We will rejoice and be glad in it"* (Psalm 118:24). We can rejoice each morning or at bedtime by listing the gifts we've experienced during the day. Be sure to jot them down in your food/blood glucose/gratitude diary. This is the wise thing to do! *"If you are wise, your wisdom will reward you"* (Proverbs 9:12).

Gratitude Words

Dr. Charles Shelton asked groups of people to select, from a list of 250 words, those they would use to best describe the opposite of feeling grateful. Five of the most commonly used words in descending order were *bitter, resentful, disappointed, dissatisfied,* and *empty.* On the other hand, the words that best described the feeling of gratitude to these groups of people in descending order were *appreciating, peaceful, love, warm,* and *inspired.*[5] That word *peaceful* is often missing when a hidden factor in diabetes management is present, and that factor is stress. Stress can have an adverse effect on blood sugar levels. We'll be examining that topic in chapter 8.

Rudyard Kipling wrote, "Words are the most powerful drug used by mankind." Someone came up with this saying: "Words are like nitroglycerine: they can blow up bridges or heal hearts." The way of wisdom also teaches the importance of what we say. *"What you say can preserve life or destroy it; so you must accept the consequences of your words"* (Proverbs 18:21). You'll be using words in your gratitude diary, words that describe interactions with others, gifts, blessings, or good things for which you are thankful! Remember to focus on the "Feel Good Page," thinking of those good things as gifts. Blessings will abound from gratitude. Try it!

The Way of Wisdom Is to Be Thankful.

"*Good news gives health to your body*" (Proverbs 15:30). "*If you really want to become wise, you must begin by having respect for the Lord. To know the Holy One is to gain understanding. Through me, you will live a long time. Years will be added to your life. If you are wise, your wisdom will reward you*" (Proverbs 9:10–12). "*Do not be anxious about anything, but in everything, by prayer and petition, with thanksgiving, present your requests to God. And the peace of God, which transcends all understanding, will guard your hearts and your minds in Christ Jesus*" (Philippians 4:6–7). "*And be thankful*" (Colossians 3:15).

---

1. Robert K. Cooper, PhD, *Flip the Switch Lose the Weight: Proven Strategies to Fuel Your Metabolism & Burn Fat 24 hours A Day* (New York: Rodale Books, 2005), 144.
2. Robert A. Emmons, *Thanks: How Practicing Gratitude Can Make You Happier* (New York: Houghton Mifflin Company, 2007), 128.
3. Emmons, 150–52.
4. Emmons, 36–37.
5. Charles M. Shelton, PhD, *The Gratitude Factor: Enhancing Your Life through Grateful Living* (Mahwah, New Jersey: HiddenSpring, 2010), 58–59, 87.

Chapter 6

Being Careful What You're Thinking and Saying, Because Your Thoughts Are Running Your Life

The news of a diagnosis of diabetes can be overwhelming. People may begin to worry about doing all the diabetes procedures correctly. They can be upset because they find they have to make too many changes. Who likes change? They may have to make changes, for example, in their eating habits and learn how carbohydrates, exercise, and medications affect blood sugar levels.

The downward pull of discouragement can occur while thinking in a negative way about the future. Let's remember what the way of wisdom states about our thinking: *"Be careful what you think, because your* thoughts run your life" (Proverbs 4:23). Have you ever caught yourself (or heard others) saying things like the following: "I did everything I was supposed to, and my blood glucose readings are still all over the place!" "I tried that new medication, and I don't feel any better." "For two months now, I've been walking regularly, but I haven't lost an ounce of weight!" "This just isn't fair; I've been doing everything I was supposed to do, and now I have to start insulin! Why have I even bothered trying?"

What Are You Saying to Yourself about Low Blood Sugars?

The newly diagnosed person with diabetes may have been told about low blood sugar or hypoglycemia and imagine how it can feel. It is one thing to think of it in an intellectual way and another to actually experience it. When the person experiences it he or she may be thinking, "This will ruin everything—my ability to drive safely and confidently as well as manage my diabetes successfully," or "Good diabetes care is now impossible. My life will be wrecked." Neither one of those statements is true. People need to learn what to do when a low blood sugar occurs—and to talk to themselves in a more pleasant, healthy way.

One of the symptoms of a low blood sugar count, or hypoglycemia, is feeling physically weaker, perhaps not having the energy to even walk. A person can also feel very hungry. If left untreated, blurry vision and incoherency can result. Hypoglycemia is a 70 mg/dl reading or less. How many grams of a quick-energy carbohydrate are needed to treat a low reading of blood glucose? A good rule of thumb is that 1 gram of glucose raises the blood sugar 3, 4, or 5 points for body weights of 200,

150, or 100 pounds, respectively. For example, 5 grams of dextrose, as found in Smarties™ or SweeTarts™ raises the blood sugar about 20 points for a 150-lb person. Most people should treat their low with about 15 grams of Smarties™ or similar candy, then wait twenty minutes and check again.[1]

It Is Nice to Have Support

In these situations, it would be good to have a support system. Sometimes people are overwhelmed with good support, whereas others are virtually on their own. The following two illustrations show the stark contrast.

One night a couple who had been married for over fifty years was lying in bed. The husband was almost asleep when he heard his wife sobbing, and he asked, "Honey, what's wrong?" "There was a time when you would give me a good night kiss before going to sleep," she said. He then gave her a kiss. He was about asleep again when his wife began to cry. "What's wrong, honey?" "There was a time when you would hold my hand before going to sleep." He then held her hand. She began to cry again when he was almost asleep. "Honey, what's wrong?" "There was a time when you would nibble on my ear before going to sleep." With that, he got right up out of bed. She said, "Honey, don't be mad, don't be mad!" He said, "Who's mad? I'm just going to get my teeth."

I like that attitude, don't you? The attitude of service can make a tremendous difference, not only to others but also to the one giving it! Wisdom's way teaches, *"Whoever refreshes others will be refreshed"* (Proverbs 11:25). According to that passage, when we are supportive in helping others with diabetes, we also help and encourage ourselves.

Now, compare that example with the following one. A doctor is talking to the wife of the patient and says, "Madam, unless you do the following, your husband isn't going to be around too long." The doctor then gave this prescription: "Make sure he gets a good, healthy breakfast every morning" (old fashioned oats and fruit etc.). "Have him come home for lunch each day, so you can feed him a low-fat, high-fiber, balanced meal. Make sure you serve him a hot supper every night, and don't burden him with any household chores." "Also," the doctor continued, "Keep the house spotless, so he's never exposed to any unnecessary germs." Later, on the way home, the husband asked his wife what the doctor had said. She paused for a moment and then said, "Honey, the doctor thinks you're not going to be around too much longer!"

The Best Support of All

There is a glaring contrast in those two situations, isn't there? Some have very supportive people in their lives, while others aren't so fortunate! What both of those examples overlooked is where the best support of all can be found. Dr. Gary Arsham puts it this way: "You are the best available source of support for living well with diabetes. You are always there and you know yourself well. No one else can take care of you as well as you can."[2]

For example, the way of wisdom states: *"The wise in heart are called discerning, and pleasant words promote instruction"* (Proverbs 16:21). Not only can pleasant words promote instruction with others, they can also promote instruction when we use them with ourselves! *"As he thinks in his heart, so is he"* (Proverbs 23:7). We can use positive thinking to our advantage! *"The tongue that brings healing is a tree of life, but a deceitful tongue crushes the spirit"* (Proverbs 15:4). We can even deceive ourselves about our future and be crushed and not healed. Instead of feeling guilty or ashamed for having diabetes, being anxious about learning all the things necessary to live well, or fearing complications, why not talk to ourselves with pleasant, encouraging words? *"Pleasant words are like honey. They are sweet to the spirit and bring healing to the body"* (Proverbs 16:24).

Positive, Upbeat Words

It's healthy to talk to ourselves with pleasant words—that is, positive, upbeat words—when facing the daily challenges of diabetes. The following way of viewing yourself by Dr. Richard Beaser of the Joslin Diabetes Center would be a pleasant, wise way to talk which I've revised as personal affirmations:

I am highly motivated and willing to perform frequent blood checks. I am basically optimistic and able to handle adversity fairly well. I am prepared to accept failure if it occurs, but also to learn and grow from it.

I think independently and make decisions with confidence, yet also have enough insight into my abilities to know my limitations and to call for help when needed. I am a strong and self-assured individual so that when monitoring or scheduling requirements affect my activities with others, I handle my needs without giving in to group pressures.

I feel comfortable with, and am able to educate those around me, about why I need to frequently check and count my carbohydrates. I feel comfortable in my ability to make appropriate adaptations so that I can participate in social activities that I enjoy.[3]

Making Comparisons with the Past

Besides talking to yourself with those affirmations, make a comparison of your situation with those in the past who faced the challenge of diabetes, but who had few of the resources we now have available today. Our thoughts, views, and actions (and, hence, confidence) will be strengthened by doing so. Which of the following two statements do you think would be the most beneficial to complete?

"I wish I was _____," or "I'm glad I'm not _____."

"I wish I was _____." Healthier, wealthier, wiser like certain others, who seemingly move along in life with no apparent challenges coming their way from diabetes? Everything seems to just smoothly pass along. Does a real feeling of gratitude or appreciation come when you think of someone like that? Or does it bring out more of a feeling of envy or resentment? It would be easy to be envious and think they have all the luck.

"I'm glad I'm not _____." I'm glad I'm not fighting a losing battle by just using the state-of-art therapy of "under-nutrition" or starvation that was available in 1919. "I'm glad I'm not: fighting a losing battle by just temporarily keeping my blood sugars down...believing that "ignorance is bliss"...making stupid decisions like... being bitter...blaming others. You can fill in the blanks. This is the approach that the apostle Paul used with the church at Thessalonica. He wrote, *"We don't want you to be ignorant about those who have died. We don't want you to grieve like other people who have no hope"* (1 Thessalonians 4:13).

Two Examples Showing a Contrast in Thinking

Two years after experiencing the eye problems I mentioned in chapter 5, I was in the hospital to have a laminectomy, or back surgery. I was recovering from the surgery in a wing of the hospital that was exclusively for those with diabetes. I was in the hospital ten days recovering, and during that time I discovered there were four people younger than me who were already blind and another person who was a little older who was blind also. I was only thirty-four.

I learned of one person, however, who was blind and only twenty-seven years old. I saw demonstrated in his life a lack of the way of wisdom principles and the devastating results that came. You could see the truth of the second half of Proverbs 10:27 in his life: *"Whoever respects the Lord will have a long life, but the life of an evil person will be cut short."* You may think *evil* is too strong of a word for this twenty-seven-year-old. It is true; I don't know what kind of support he had growing up with his diabetes or what kinds of friends he had. I was blessed with loving parents who helped me manage my diabetes, as well as good friends.

I learned that he had been in and out of the hospital with diabetic ketoacidosis, a condition that results from the lack of insulin for an extended period, which creates very elevated blood glucose levels. This results in a toxic method of metabolizing food for energy, resulting in a concentration of free fatty acids, dehydration, loss of fluid (which brings loss of electrolytes like potassium, chloride, and sodium), and an increase in counter-regulatory hormones like glucagon and cortisol. This is a serious condition that can lead to coma. A person in this condition must have an infusion of electrolytes, insulin, and some glucose as a proper source of energy.[4] All of this had apparently been happening with this young man. He had already been there for days when I was in the hospital.

He blamed anything and everyone for his situation instead of accepting responsibility! The way of wisdom teaches: *"A man's spirit* (cheerful heart or will to live) *sustains him in sickness, but a crushed spirit who can bear?"* (Proverbs 18:14). Instead of using the button at his bed to summon a nurse, he would rave like a madman. Sometimes he would also bang on the wall while ranting—it happened to be the wall that separated our rooms. When a nurse came into his room to help, he would lambaste her for not coming sooner. All of this wouldn't have had to happen, if he had just learned to use the principles we are examining in this book. The way of wisdom teachings are for health and well-being. *"Listen, my son, accept what I say, and the years of your life will be many. I guide you in the way of wisdom and lead you along straight paths. When you walk, your steps will not be hampered; when you run, you will not stumble....My son, pay attention to what I say; listen closely to my words. Do not let them out of your sight, keep them within your heart; for they are life to those who find them and health to a man's whole body"* (Proverbs 4:10–12,20–22).

Contrast of Twenty-Seven-Year-Old with Elizabeth Hughes

Back to our fill in the blank statement, "I'm glad I'm not _____," that is, like that twenty-seven-year-old in the room next to me in Trinity Lutheran Hospital. A better example is that of Elizabeth Hughes. She was diagnosed with diabetes at the age of eleven and spent the next four years on the "under-nutrition, starvation therapy" prescribed by Dr. Frederick Allen. We can be thankful that we don't have to go through what she experienced. We can also see, however, important characteristics she had that we should emulate. It was her focus on good things in very difficult circumstances that helped her to live through the pain and hunger she faced. She used the pleasant words and gratitude principles, as displayed in her letters to her mother.

Economic status did not exempt people from being diagnosed with diabetes then, just as it doesn't now. Her father, Charles Hughes, had been the governor of New York; he went on to hold various offices, like the United States Secretary of State under the Harding administration and later a Supreme Court Justice. When she was diagnosed in 1918 at the age of eleven, she was five feet tall and weighed seventy-five pounds. When Dr. Frederick Banting, the discoverer of insulin, examined her on August 16, 1922, which was three days before her fifteenth birthday, she weighed forty-five pounds.

After being diagnosed, her parents were able to hire a nurse, Blanche Burgess, to help her. She had been trained by Dr. Elliott Joslin of Boston. Ultimately, however, as was previously mentioned, the best available source of support for managing diabetes is from the one who has it. She would have to learn and adhere to what was required for her to live. She had learned self-control and discipline from her parents, which helped her tremendously.

The way of wisdom states: *"Like a city whose walls are broken through is a person who lacks self-control"* (Proverbs 25:28). A defense mechanism for cities in ancient times was their walls, which protected them from enemy armies. The wise state that our defense is self-control, which can be used against onslaughts of eating too much delicious food, sitting too much, or just giving up on following a healthy plan. It is interesting how Elizabeth's self-control was reinforced by her focus, by what she was writing and saying about her daily life.

There were times during the next four years, after being diagnosed with diabetes, that she consumed as little as four hundred calories per day. By the spring of 1921, she only weighed fifty-two pounds. She could only eat a mundane diet of food that kept her from showing sugar in her urine. As her father was the Secretary of State, their home for a time was in Washington, DC. It was in that environment of political stress that she could not attain proper control. They could not keep an environment of peace and calm there for her; there was just too much activity. Her parents made the decision to send her for six months to the island of Bermuda, accompanied by her nurse.

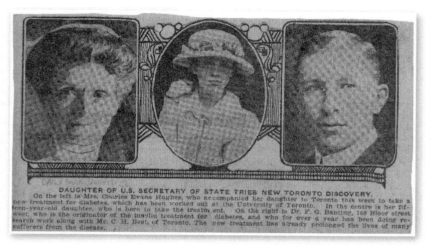

DAUGHTER OF U.S. SECRETARY OF STATE TRIES NEW TORONTO DISCOVERY.
On the left is Mrs. Charles Evans Hughes who accompanied her daughter to Toronto this week to take a new treatment for diabetes, which has been worked out at the University of Toronto. In the centre is her fifteen-year-old daughter, who is here to take the treatment. On the right is Dr. F. G. Banting, 160 Bloor street west, who is the originator of the insulin treatment for diabetes, and who for over a year has been doing research work along with Mr. C H. Best, of Toronto. The new treatment has already prolonged the lives of many sufferers from the disease.

Elizabeth Hughes before receiving insulin. Image courtesy of the Thomas Fisher Rare Book Library, University of Toronto.

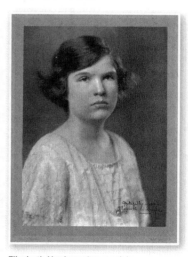

Elizabeth Hughes after receiving insulin, about 1923 Photo courtesy of the Thomas Fisher Rare Book Library, University of Toronto.v

She loved to write to her mother during her stay, and it is interesting what she decided to write about. She could have written about her intense sense of hunger and weakness, but there would be little new to say about that. Instead her letters were an upbeat recounting of her days. After researching her letters, Catherine Cox wrote, "She might have been writing cheerful letters because that was what she wanted to receive....She kept her letters focused on the positive and downplayed the inconveniences of her condition....It is also possible that with her upbeat tone she was just trying to think positively."[5]

Of course, Elizabeth Hughes was one of the fortunate ones to receive some of the first doses of insulin. She described it as, "Oh, it is simply too wonderful for words this stuff."[6] She died in 1981, after taking 42,000 injections of insulin over a span of fifty-eight years!

Choose the Color

A sympathetic friend said to a crippled woman, "Affliction does so color life." "Yes," the woman replied, "but I propose to choose the color." Isn't that what Elizabeth did? She chose her attitude. The way of wisdom states: *"The will to live can get you through sickness, but no one can live with a broken spirit,"* or, translated differently, *"A man's spirit sustains him in sickness, but a crushed spirit who can bear?"* (Proverbs 18:14).

When the apostle Paul was in prison, he wrote this advice to the Philippians: *"Finally, my brothers and sisters, always think about what is true. Think about what is noble, right and pure. Think about what is lovely and worthy of respect. If anything is excellent or worthy of praise, think about those kinds of things"* (Philippians 4:8). He is pointing out that we can choose how to think. This is God's way of wisdom. Endurance and better health comes by focusing on the good news! *"A cheerful look brings joy to your heart. And good news gives health to your body"* (Proverbs 15:30).

In summary, have great expectations of yourself. Use the affirmations mentioned in this chapter to develop healthy, pleasant self-talk. Compare yourself with those in the past by using this phrase: "I'm glad I'm not _____." Realize what advantages you have available today. Remember these two phrases from the way of wisdom: *"Pleasant words are like honey. They*

are sweet to the spirit and bring healing to the body"
(Proverbs 16:24), and *"If you are wise; your wisdom will reward you"* (Proverbs 9:12).

---

1. John Walsh, PA, CDE, *Using Insulin: Everything You Need for Success with Insulin* (San Diego: Torrey Pines Press, 2003), 220.
2. Gary Arsham, MD, and Ernest Lowe, *Diabetes: A Guide to Living Well* (Alexandria, Virginia: American Diabetes Association, 2004), 15.
3. Richard Beaser, MD, *Outsmarting Diabetes: A Dynamic Approach for Reducing the Effects of Insulin-Dependent Diabetes* (Minneapolis: Chronimed Publishing, 1994) 151–52.
4. Richard Beaser, MD, ed., *Joslin Diabetes Deskbook: A Guide for Primary Care Providers* (Boston: Joslin Diabetes Center, 2010), 420–31.
5. Catherine Cox, *The Fight to Survive* (New York: Kaplan Publishing, 2009), 113–14.
6. Michael Bliss, *The Discovery of Insulin* (Chicago: The University of Chicago Press, 1982), 152.

Part 2

....

Doing The Things
We Need To Do

Chapter 7

Helping Others up a Hill Will Help You Get to the Summit as Well: Encourage Others and Be Encouraged

Some people have the viewpoint that diabetes is "my personal disease, and I'm ashamed I have it. I'm certainly not going to let others know that I have it. If I do tell, the people who think it is their solemn duty to scrutinize what I do, the diabetes police, will be asking things like 'should you really be eating that?'" That's one way to think of it; however, there is a completely different perspective that, when used properly, will encourage you while you actually encourage others. It is based upon the wisdom teaching that says *"Whoever refreshes others will be refreshed"* (Proverbs 11:25). How does this principle of refreshing others actually refresh the one who gives? Let me give two examples—one where you feel energized, enthused, and healthy; and one where you're not in the mood or just don't feel well. Then we'll make a practical application to managing diabetes.

Helping Others When You Feel Well

Several years ago I was helping a church do a survey door-to-door, talking to people in the neighborhood about topics that could be used for seminars to help people in day-to-day living. I came to one house where an older gentleman came to the door. I told him what we were doing and showed him a list of topics like family enrichment, stress management, money management, feeling good about yourself, and so on.

He looked at the list and thought some of the topics were interesting. "When we have a lecture on one of these topics, we would sure like to have you come," I said. He said he wouldn't be able to, because his wife was confined in the house. I asked him if one of his children could come and stay with her. He said, "We've been married over fifty years, and we don't have any children." I asked if maybe a friend could come over and stay with her. He replied, "We don't have any friends. In fact, no one cares about us!"

Several weeks later the church started a "Meals-on-Wheels" program. I remembered the man and went to see if he and his wife would like to participate and receive a warm meal several times a week. He was reluctant; he didn't want anyone coming into the house. I explained that the food could be brought to the porch, and no one would have to come in. He still hesitated. I then told him how delicious and warm the food would be. He finally agreed. As I was walking down off the porch, he said something. I couldn't hear him, so I said, "Pardon me?" He repeated, "You've really lifted me up!" Well, I was the one who was really lifted up. I practically floated back to the car. Yes, it is true: *"Whoever refreshes others will be refreshed"* (Proverbs 11:25).

Years later I heard the rest of the story. The church continued to take meals to him and care for him, even after his wife died, and because he had been helped so much over the years, he wanted to show his appreciation by leaving what he had to them at the end of his life!

Helping Others When You Just Don't Feel Well

A southern California pastime of whale watching has developed when the gray whales migrate. Author Dave Grant tells about going to see them. He says some people became seasick. It's been said that with seasickness, you have two fears: the first is that you're going to die, and the second is that you're not going to die.

Suppose a person is seasick, and I come up and say, "I don't mean to bother you, but I've really got a bad headache. Do you have an aspirin?" Can you imagine how that person might respond? "Go away, don't bother me," or "can't you see I'm sick?" I could go away thinking, *That guy is sure selfish. He's all wrapped up in himself.* It's hard to think of someone else's needs when you're overwhelmed with your own. But suppose that person's own grandchild falls overboard. What would happen to the seasickness? In most cases it would disappear because of a greater need. Remember, *"Whoever refreshes others will be refreshed"* (Proverbs 11:25). We can help ourselves by helping others![1]

Some people seem to become so-called experts when they hear someone has diabetes, thinking they know everything about it. After all, they may have had a relative who had diabetes, and they know all the weaknesses they had in not managing it. This can make others reluctant to tell them they have diabetes. That's one way to view having the disease—but if you let others know, couldn't you better educate them? When others know you have diabetes, they may actually reveal they have it too, giving you an opportunity to encourage them. You may be thinking, however, that you actually don't know that much yourself.

"What Do You Know That We Don't Know?"

It is true that we all have more to learn. Even the wise have more to learn, according to the introduction of the Proverbs: *"...let the wise listen and add to their learning, and let the discerning get guidance"* (Proverbs 1:5). In the biblical book of Job, there is one phrase that indicates Eliphaz, a friend of Job, may have thought he knew more than he actually did: *"What do you know that we do not know? What insights do you have that we do not have?"* (Job 15:9). Here is Eliphaz, healthy, wealthy, and wise, talking to his friend who has just lost all ten of his grown children in what sounds like a tornado. Job's grieving wife has been driven to despair; his health is now gone, replaced with excruciating pain; and his status in life is completely changed with the loss of his wealth, the loss of just about everything he has; and he now feels alienated from God. And now this wealthy, healthy, wise man, Eliphaz, asks, "What do you know that we don't know?" Do you get the picture? What Eliphaz does not know is called *what*

Job is experiencing! The diabetes police may think they know a lot, but they don't know from personal experience what it's like to live every day with diabetes.

There is plenty for us to learn from our own experiences and from those of others. It might be in the very suffering we experience that we'll become better equipped to serve, to help others who suffer, and thus help ourselves! "What do you know that we don't know?" You may know a lot that we don't know! "To tell or not to tell?" is the question. If we keep our diabetes a secret, we will never know the benefits we may experience with others, learning from them as well as helping them. Again, the way of wisdom teaches that *"Whoever refreshes others will be refreshed"* (Proverbs 11:25).

Helping and Understanding

A teaching for healthy living that relates to this is found in Proverbs 3:3–4: *"Never let loyalty and kindness get away from you! Wear them like a necklace; write them deep within your heart. Then you will find favor and good understanding, in the sight of God and people."* This relates to the words given in the previous verse: *"... for they will prolong your life many years and bring you peace and prosperity"* (Proverbs 3:2). Loyalty with kindness to others benefits not only those receiving it but also those giving it. Someone once said to me, "You've really made a difference in my life." When he told me that, I really hadn't thought my help with his diabetes had made such a significant difference in his life, but to my surprise it had! "Would you be willing to visit my son [who had Type 1 diabetes] in the hospital?" I was surprised to have that question asked, but answered with

"Of course, I'll visit him! To give encouragement was a reason for starting a diabetes support group," I said.

"Ever since I met you, things have gone so much better for me," said another person. I initially met this person, Randy, in the hospital after the certified diabetes educator requested that I come visit him. He was non-compliant, putting sheets over his head when health care providers tried to teach and help him. But since I had had diabetes since I was seven, and he since he was about thirteen, he opened up to me. He was about thirty-three at that time. He eventually ended up being on peritoneal kidney dialysis. He also was put on a transplant list and, months later, received a kidney and pancreas. Then a few months later, he was involved in a train/car wreck, breaking numerous ribs, his arm, and femur, and sustaining severe trauma to his head. He made the statement "Ever since I met you things have gone so much better for me," after being in rehab for months. But ever since I met him, he had been learning about God's love and way of wisdom, and that knowledge was making a real difference in his life!

A person called me whom I hadn't seen or heard from in more than a year, because I had moved out of state. In the past, before I moved, we would have weekly meetings at a food court and discuss our diabetes management. He invited me to also be on his bowling league team, but eventually we stopped meeting for our diabetes management. A year later he called while in the hospital. He had to have a toe amputated and have reconstruction surgery on his heel because of diabetes complications. I empathetically listened to him and encouraged him to stay vigilant, so he could outsmart diabetes. I told him he could turn everything around and feel better. Again, I didn't know I had made such an impact on his life that he wanted to talk to me from another state a year after seeing him last! On the phone he became so emotional he couldn't contain his tears and began sobbing. All these are comments and examples from people that I've met and helped through diabetes support groups I've facilitated.

Starting Diabetes Support Groups

Every single person needs the way of wisdom principles to outsmart diabetes, whether he or she knows it or not. One principle that was useful for me is the one found in Proverbs 11:25, which I keep emphasizing—*"Whoever refreshes others will be refreshed."* In other words, it is the principle of support and service. When it comes to outsmarting diabetes, we all need help! During the last fifty years, I've received help from my parents, my wife, and some outstanding doctors along the way. In the first grade, I spent several days of my Christmas vacation in the hospital before being dismissed on Christmas Eve, 1960. When I woke up the next day, I was excited—after all, it was Christmas, and there were presents. The day held a different kind of excitement when my dad said, "Kenny, it's time for your shot." He had to chase me all over the house. Of course, I've been taking insulin ever since.

For the next twenty years, I accepted the disease by casually watching my diet, taking my shots, and checking my urine for sugar. I would often miss school on Mondays, pretending that I was sick. But in reality I probably was sick with high blood sugars. I didn't really take diabetes serious until after being married for five years, then going to graduate school, and finally going to an in-depth, weeklong education class in the hospital. I also received my first glucose meter, an Ames, in 1981.

Service and support was given to me when I was first diagnosed and admitted to the hospital on December 20, 1960. People continued to serve and help me in the following years. Finally, after having diabetes for more than thirty years, I thought I might have experienced and learned enough to be able to encourage others, but since then I've learned you can start helping others almost immediately.

Starting in 1992, I decided to help others to meet this challenge by starting a diabetes support group at Good Samaritan Hospital in Kearney, Nebraska, with the help of Dr. Richard Hranac. I was able to meet, serve, and encourage hundreds of people over the next few years, and I continue to do so wherever I live. I believe encouraging others has been one of the important keys for me to manage my diabetes for the last twenty-five years. Also, being grateful for all the tools available, including educational resources that were scarce twenty years ago, has also helped me to manage my diabetes, instead of letting it manage me! The way of wisdom principles that we are examining have been there all along to use. They are the real keys for the management of diabetes, because they come from God!

Loyalty, Kindness, and Understanding

As the wisdom teaching instructs, one is to have loyalty and kindness toward others. *"Never let loyalty and kindness get away from you!"* (Proverbs 3:3) Who can have this loyalty and kindness, which results in good understanding, better than those facing many of the same challenges themselves? It's one thing for a doctor to tell a woman to check her blood glucose twice a day instead of once, when he doesn't even have to check his at all. On the other hand, when you have to check yourself several times a day, and you encourage someone to be more vigilant about checking theirs, it can make a difference.

Instead of Putting People in Their Place, Put Yourself in Their Place. Lift People Up, Don't Put People Down. If Discouraged, Encourage!

From your own experience, you have a better emotional understanding about what others are feeling and facing. To tell or not to tell others about their own diabetes is a concern that some people have. When people let their diabetes be their own personal, private disease, however, they miss out on helping others and thus being encouraged and in better control themselves. Notice what the way of wisdom teaches about helping others in the following passages: *"A good person gives life to others; the wise person teaches others how to live"* (Proverbs 11:30). *"Generous people will be blessed, because they share their food with the poor"* (Proverbs 22:9).

What does wisdom instruct will happen to those who follow these teachings? *"Blessed is the one who finds wisdom. Blessed is the one who gains understanding. Wisdom pays better than silver does. She earns more than gold does. She is worth more than rubies. Nothing you want can compare with her"* (Proverbs 3:13-15). Those who follow these instructions are blessed and nothing a person desires will compare to finding and using wisdom.

Notice what is stated in Proverbs 19:17. *"Those who are kind to the poor lend to the LORD, and he will* reward them for what they have done." When we help those in need it is as though we are lending what we have to the Lord and he always pays back what we give with interest. It is like what Jesus taught when he said, "Give, and it will be given to you. A good measure, pressed down, shaken together and running over, will be poured into your lap. For with the measure you use, it will be measured to you" (Luke 6:38). How does this happen? Since wisdom is far superior than silver, gold or rubies the results are far more valuable too.

One woman's mother was in the hospital with cancer. She wanted to do something very special for her so she bought a very expensive nightgown with matching robe for her to wear. At least she would be the prettiest dressed woman in the hospital she thought.

She brought the packaged gift with some apprehension to her hospital room. Her mother had grown up during the depression and as a result she was very frugal and was opposed to waste of any kind. So when she opened the gift for a long time she just sat there and said nothing. Her daughter wasn't surprised when her mother finally said, "Would you mind returning it to the store? I don't really want it." Instead she pointed to a newspaper display ad she had opened on her bed. "This is what I really want, if you could get that," she said. It was a display advertisement of very expensive summer designer purses.

The daughter's first thought, and she herself was a medical doctor, was that she won't even be around in the spring much less the summer to use it. It was January and she didn't think she would even live through the spring. Then she realized that her mother, in her own subtle way, was actually asking her if she believed she would still be alive in six months. Once she realized this she immediately took the gown back and bought her the purse. "That was many years ago. The purse is worn out and long gone, as are at least half a dozen others," she wrote.[2] What she was doing was following wisdom's way. The results were far more valuable than any silver, gold or rubies, weren't they?

Wisdom teaches us to project hope, be understanding and give encouragement to those who are in need. *"Whenever you are able, do good to people who need help. If you have what your neighbor asks for, don't say, "Come back later. I will give it to you tomorrow"* (Proverbs 3:27-28). What we often have is a kind word or some act of encouragement, which can bolster someone's attitude and help them deal with a difficult situation. And when we do, we too will be blessed! *"A generous person will prosper; whoever refreshes others will be refreshed"* (Proverbs 11:25). *"Those who are kind reward themselves, but the cruel do themselves harm"* (Proverbs 11:17).

Research on Giving Support

A survey of 4,500 American adult volunteers was done in 2010, with 68 percent of those surveyed stating that volunteering helped them feel physically healthier. In addition, 89 percent of the volunteers reported that volunteering had given them a greater sense of well-being, and 73 percent felt it had lowered their stress levels.[3]

Other research also reveals that when people give of their time, talent, and treasure in volunteer work, the result is that they are healthier. The healthy thing to do is to encourage others. A 2005 study done by researchers at Stanford University revealed that volunteering was a powerful protector of mental and physical health. The study was called the Longitudinal Study of Aging and consisted of more than 7500 people who were over age seventy. Volunteering was shown to be healthy, and those who frequently did so benefited the most.[4]

Someone could ask, "Which comes first, the generosity or good health?" After all, healthier people can volunteer more. One hundred thirty-seven multiple sclerosis (MS) patients were divided into three groups. Two groups were either given eight weeks of coping skills training or received phone calls from other MS patients, who had been trained to listen and give support. Those who were taught to compassionately listen were the third group, which was smaller. This group's members improved their outlook and health even more than the others. Here we have people who were already ill, and yet, giving bolstered their emotional and physical well-being more than receiving.[5]

Jesus taught, *"It is more blessed to give than to receive"* (Acts 20:35). Here is another example of how this principle works. When AT&T was broken up into the "baby Bells," in the early 1980s a study of a subsidiary of AT&T—Illinois Bell, which was downsized from 26,000 to 14,000—was done. The study was done on 450 of the managers to see how the stress affected their health. Under the stress of the situation, two-thirds of the managers ended up with heart attacks, strokes, ulcers, arthritis, or cancer. The other third were the "hardy" ones, who seemed to be stress resistant. One of the qualities found in this group, however, was their commitment to do their best while also helping others through this difficult time.[5] Many studies have been done since that time, some of which have already been mentioned, that show volunteering to help others is a protector to mental and physical health.

Many people are struggling and need encouragement. What is most important is not making sure as few people as possible know you have diabetes, but rather encouraging those who have it. That is one of the healthy things we can do. The way of wisdom states, *"The generous will themselves be blessed"* and *"A generous person will prosper; whoever refreshes others will be refreshed"* (Proverbs 22:9, 11:25).

Diabetes Support Groups

God's wisdom teaches to *"not make friends with the hot-tempered, do not associate with those who are easily angered, or you may learn their ways and get yourself ensnared"* (Proverbs 22:24–25). The way of wisdom also teaches, *"Whoever walks with the wise grows wise"* (Proverbs 13:20). When we attend a diabetes support group, we are joining people who can lift us up, not tear us down; encourage us, not discourage us! We all desire the same thing—to live better with diabetes, feeling better and being healthier.

One woman at our diabetes support group knew she needed to start walking, but she also knew she needed the support of others to get started. She asked if there was anyone who could meet at the park at a certain time to walk. Can you imagine how it would be to show up to walk and have about a dozen others there to help you get started? It would be inspiring, encouraging, and motivating, wouldn't it? And it was motivating! I've discovered that when I look for people I can encourage and support, they've helped me too! Those who showed up to help her get started walking, walked too. So in a sense, she was helping them, also. When we look for others to support, we too will be blessed!

1. Dave Grant, *The Ultimate Power* (Old Tappan, New Jersey: Fleming H. Revell Company, 1983), 123.

2. Bernie S. Siegel, MD, *Peace, Love & Healing: Bodymind Communication & The Path to Self-healing: An Exploration* (New York: Harper & Row, Publishers, 1989), 17-18.

3. Stephen G. Post, PhD, *The Hidden Gifts of Helping: How the Power of Giving, Compassion, and Hope Can Get Us through Hard Times* (San Francisco: Jossey-Bass, 2011), 32.

4. Stephen G. Post, PhD, *Why Good Things Happen to Good People: The Exciting New Research That Proves the Link between Doing Good and Living a Longer, Healthier, Happier Life* (New York: Broadway Books, 2007), 68. Post, 55.

5. Al Siebert, PhD, *The Resiliency Advantage: Master Change, Thrive Under Pressure, and Bounce Back from Setbacks* (San Francisco: Berret-Koehler Publishers, Inc., 2005), 41–42.

Chapter 8

Managing Diabetes Perfectly Doesn't Equal Perfect Results: How to Effectively Cope with the Hidden Factor of Stress

Someone says, "Yesterday I followed my exercise and meal plan almost perfectly! So I woke up this morning and my blood sugar was 300, which is ridiculous! Why should I even bother trying?" People can easily get down on themselves, thinking they are doing everything they possibly can and still not be in control. They can get stressed out about all kinds of circumstances and not be at peace.

Just having diabetes can generate stressful events, like remembering to take your medications each day at the proper time. Having high blood sugars that result in becoming dehydrated, having no energy, and making repeated trips to the restroom becomes frustrating and annoying. The struggle with keeping blood sugars in a normal range, especially when eating out, is a struggle. Coping with the anxiety that comes from low blood sugars, and properly handling the lows when they come, can be one of the most stressful events. If you've ever been so low in blood sugar that you feel like you're on the brink of passing out, and you're trying to squeeze every ounce or even milligram of energy remaining to keep from passing out, then you know how stressful it can be!

How Does the Stress of Conflict (or Stress, Period) Affect Your Blood Glucose?

Have you ever checked your blood glucose and discovered for some unforeseen reason you are sky-high? You try to eliminate all possible reasons. You don't have a cold or infection, to your knowledge; you counted your carbohydrates and ate a healthy meal; you took just the right amount of medication; but none of these seem to be giving you the answer. What could the answer be? Could it be stress?

We can bring stressful situations onto ourselves. While sitting in a large waiting room to see my doctor, I noticed a couple who had become impatient. It was true that usually this doctor would get behind on appointments, which, I've discovered over the years, did not make him unusual in any way. This happens quite often. We shouldn't even be surprised when it happens. I would usually bring something to read or study, expecting to stay awhile. Apparently, this couple felt they had waited long enough. I heard the husband say to his wife that if the nurse didn't call her name by the top of the hour, he would go get their car. The time came without hearing her name, so he went out in a huff to get their car. When she saw him drive up, she got up and left, too. Within one minute after that, I heard the nurse call for them, but they were gone. I heard the nurse say to the receptionist that she was sure she had seen her. If they had just waited a minute, they would have heard her name called. To them, this was a stressful situation, and it could have easily resulted in an elevated blood glucose level.

At another doctor's waiting room, I came expecting a long wait. I started reading a very interesting book, and all of a sudden the doctor himself, Dr. Richard Hellman, came out to greet me. I expressed my surprise about being called so quickly and that I was prepared to wait much longer, as I was in the middle of reading a very intriguing book. Then he said in a humorous way, "When we saw people bringing sleeping bags, we decided something had to be done about the long waits."

A study was done of a person with Type 1 diabetes, who was connected to a continuous glucose monitor. One day his blood glucose range was from 105 to 150, which was very good. The next day his activities were very similar, with one exception—he went to a soccer game. He started the game at a normal range, but once the game started, his level began to rise and peaked at 302. He hadn't had anything to eat for several hours. His rapid increase in blood sugar was a result of stress. He may have been caught up in the game, thinking his team might lose.[1]

What Normally Happens to Blood Sugars With Too Much Stress

When there is a rapid increase in blood glucose, it is also important to consider activities and even concerns or worries one may have about work, family, and finances. When we perceive something as a threat or as stressful, like a conflict with someone, the brain recognizes the danger and releases an array of stress hormones like cortisol, epinephrine, and norepineph-rine.[2] The epinephrine puts the body on alert, and the cortisol provides the body with protein for energy production (gluconeogenesis) by converting amino acids into usable carbohydrates (glucose) in the liver. Also, a resistance to insulin can occur, causing a greater need for available insulin.[3] The end result of stress can be an increase in blood glucose levels. Peace or calm is what is needed in stressful situations.

Peace and Calm

How can the way of wisdom help in stressful situations? When wisdom's way is followed, a more peaceful, composed lifestyle can result. *"My child, do not forget my teaching, but let your heart keep my commandments; for length of days and years of life and abundant welfare they will give you"* (Proverbs 3:1–2). Another Bible translation puts it the following way: *"My son, do not forget my teaching, but keep my commands in your heart, for they will prolong your life many years and bring you peace and prosperity."*

There are three benefits that stand out in this reading: a longer life, peace, and abundant welfare. In this case, the word *peace* can mean completeness or wholeness, and *prosperity* can mean abundant welfare. When a person puts this wisdom into practice, like the father instructs his son to do, then peace and abundant welfare can result. This peace will be with God, a calming peace within oneself, and in relationships with others. Conflict with others contributes to stress, which can directly affect your blood sugar control and, thus, your management of diabetes!

"When She Came Crawling to Me on Her Hands and Knees..."

There was a man telling his friend that he and his wife had a serious argument the night before. "But it ended," he said, "when she came crawling to me on her hands and knees." "What did she say?" asked the friend. The husband replied, "She said, 'Come out from under that bed, you coward!'" That's a humorous story, but in real life there is often tension in relationships at work, family, or with friends that can cause havoc to blood sugar levels.

Some people talk as though they are experts on diabetes, telling you what you need to do. You know they know very little about it. It would be easy to be insulted and put them in their place and let the stress grow, but the way of wisdom says *"the prudent overlook an insult"* (Proverbs 12:16). Another stressful situation could be when you are unjustly criticized for something you know is not your fault, and you are ready to harshly set the accuser straight! The way of wisdom, however, would instruct you that *"A gentle answer turns away wrath, but a harsh word stirs up anger"* (Proverbs 15:1).

"If your enemy is hungry, give him food to eat; if he is thirsty, give him water to drink. In doing this, you will heap burning coals on his head, and the LORD will reward you. (Proverbs 25:21-22).

In other words, this kind of response is totally unexpected and can cause a person to be uncomfortable.

The way of wisdom teaches one to have the right perspective about people. When people don't have the perspective toward others that God's wisdom teaches, then "be yourself" is about the worst advice one could give someone. Have you noticed how selfish, bitter, and harsh some people can be? If a person is like that, you don't want to say "be yourself," do you? A good question for some people is, "Do I hurt people, or am I too easily hurt by them?" If the answer is yes to either part of the question, then again, blood sugar levels will be adversely affected because of the tension and stress in relationships. There are many instructions or commands to put into practice. They will be very helpful to remember and use in difficult situations.

It's Nice to Be Important, But It Is More Important to Be Nice

One of the way of wisdom's teachings deals with how we speak to others. *"The heart of a righteous person carefully considers* (ponder, meditate) *how to answer, but the mouths of wicked people pour out a flood of evil things"* (Proverbs 15:28). Also, wisdom teaches us to put into practice the following instructions: *"The wise in heart are called discerning, and pleasant words promote instruction"* (Proverbs 16:21). *"Pleasant words are like honey. They are sweet to the spirit and bring healing to the body"* (Proverbs 16:24). *"An anxious heart weighs a man down, but a kind word cheers him up"* (Proverbs 12:25). So instead of getting cross to get your thoughts across, it is much better to be gentle, pleasant, and kind. In fact, Proverbs 25:15 says, *"With patience you can convince a ruler, and a gentle word can get through to the hard-headed."*

Another teaching instructs us to avoid focusing with jealousy on what others have. Proverbs 14:30 states, *"Peace of mind means a healthy body, but jealousy will rot your bones."* So peace contributes to prolonging one's life by alleviating the stress and worry one may feel within and the tension one can experience interacting with others.

You Can't Get Ahead by Getting Even; Instead, Overlook Insults and Offenses

---

Other important wisdom teachings that help in managing stress include the following: *"A person's wisdom* (i.e., God's wisdom) *yields patience; it is to one's glory to overlook an offense"* (Proverbs 19:11). *"A fool shows his annoyance at once, but a prudent man overlooks an insult"* (Proverbs 12:16). *"Anyone who is patient has great understanding. But anyone who gets angry quickly shows how foolish he is"* (Proverbs 14:29). *"A fool gives full vent to his anger, but a wise man keeps himself under control"* (Proverbs 29:11). This wisdom to overlook offenses and insults, to be patient and self-controlled, is for our benefit. *"They are the key to life for those who find them; they bring health to the whole body"* (Proverbs 4:22). Also Keep the following in mind: *"If you are wise, your wisdom will reward you"* (Proverbs 9:12).

Cover over Offenses, Instead of Telling About Them Again and Again

---

An example that shows how practical these instructions are comes from the following research of a hundred engineers. These engineers, who had recently been laid off, were studied to learn the effects expressing or venting their anger would have on their welfare. The researchers divided them into three groups. In the first group, the questions asked were probing for hostility toward the company, like "How has the company been unfair to you?" In the second group, the questions were probing for hostility toward supervisors, like "How could your supervisor have prevented your layoff?" The third group had questions that were neutral, like "What is your opinion of the technical library?" Those discussing the wrongs in the first two groups became much angrier after venting their anger than those who were in the third group; those people did not have the opportunity to vent anger, because of the type of questions asked. Many other research studies have reached the same conclusion—that hashing and rehashing anger does not release it; on the contrary, it rekindles it, reinforces it, and reaffirms it.[4] Hostility contributes to underlying chronic stress and thus health. Some of the signs and symptoms of chronic stress are general irritability, easily fatigued, depression, loss of appetite, anxiety, nervousness, chronic muscle pains and insomnia.

When it comes to rekindling hostility over offenses, the way of wisdom teaches the opposite. Instead of venting one's anger, repeating offenses over and over again, the way of wisdom teaches to cover them over and give love an opportunity to grow. It is put this way in Proverbs 17:9: *"He who covers over an offense promotes love, but whoever repeats the matter separates close friends."*

Sometimes circumstances present themselves where a person may not even feel stressed, but an elevated blood sugar check later reveals the presence of stress. After all factors are eliminated stress is the answer in those situations. There are other times when one obviously feels stress. Some of the symptoms of acute stress are pounding heart, rapid pulse, trembling, shaky, dry throat and mouth, change in blood sugar level, sweating, diarrhoea or frequent urination, indigestion and tension headache.[5] I began to experience that pounding heart, rapid pulse and tension in a class I was teaching. It was caused by a potential outbreak of volatile hostility between two individuals in the class. Instead of an outbreak of anger, however, I saw wisdom vividly put into practice by these two men.

Doug and Ernie

I was about to teach a class on a Sunday morning, and a new student named Doug was sitting next to me. Just as the class session was about to begin, in walked Ernie on the other side of the classroom. Doug leaned over to me and, looking at Ernie, asked me if he was Ernie...giving his full name. I said it was, and he then quickly told me that several years earlier, he had been accused of the manslaughter of Ernie's uncle. The case went to trial, and the trial had to be moved to a different part of the state. He was eventually acquitted.

Ernie had already been an active member of the class and continued to learn more and more of the way of wisdom. So what do you think happened after class? Did he just abruptly walk out of the class? Did he come up to Doug and say something demeaning and offensive? No, when class was over, he simply came over to Doug and shook his hand, welcoming him to class and thus using the wisdom principle of overlooking an offense. If either of them had had diabetes, their blood sugar levels might have been spiking sky-high during the class, because of the anxiety they would be experiencing—the tense, sick feeling in their stomachs.

It would not, however, been relieved like it was if there had been bitterness and resentment embedded within their thinking. I was just a bystander observing, having a tense feeling throughout the class and my blood sugar most likely did spike up! Thankfully wisdom was used, bringing relief to a tense situation.

Even when you anticipate a tense situation like making a phone call concerning a conflict or important matter with someone, you can use techniques to relieve stress. One technique is to use "a mind-escape word or phrase." Choose a word that is comforting to you like *"God is my shield"* (Proverbs 30:5-6). Breath slowly and deeply while sitting in a comfortable position. As you are sitting focus on the air as it is going in and out. Think of yourself in a relaxed situation. It could be outdoors or inside, on a rainy or sunshiny day and then begin to repeat your mind-escape word or phrase. A similar technique is to divert your attention from the tension. According to Frank Ghinassi, PhD, instructor in psychiatry at Harvard Medical School, "Changing your thoughts can give you immediate control over how you respond to stress."[6]

According to Proverbs 22:17-19, we build trust in God when we have his wisdom entrenched in our memory. *"Pay attention and listen to the sayings of the wise; apply your heart to what I teach, for it is pleasing when you keep them in your heart and have all of them ready on your lips. So that your trust may be in the LORD, I teach you today, even you"* (Proverbs 22:17-19). Another passage says, *"Get wisdom, get understanding; do not forget my words or swerve from them. Do not forsake wisdom, and she will protect you; love her, and she will watch over you"* (Proverbs 4:5-6). One reason to have these teachings in your memory is put this way in Proverbs 4:23: *"Be careful what you think, because your thoughts run your life"* (Proverbs 4:23).

It is our focus that can make a difference! *"He who seeks good finds goodwill, but evil comes to him who searches for it"* (Proverbs 11:27). Consider the following mind-escape phrases to use when facing stressful situations: God is my *"fortified tower"* (Proverbs 18:10) or *"secure fortress"* (Proverbs 14:26).

Many times during a stressful situation when patience is needed, I've repeated to myself that *"the patient have great understanding,"* which comes from Proverbs 14:29. Repeating a passage like that gives a sense of relaxation and control. Have you ever felt like lashing out at someone and making the best speech you will ever regret? If you have, think *"he who holds his tongue is wise"* (Proverbs 10:19)! Being understanding and wise is how we all want to be considered. Repeating passages like those in tense situations will actually help us to be that way!

Four More Practical Ways to Counter the Effects of Stress on Health and Well-Being

---

Movement: Movement is one way to counter the physical effects of stress. The levels of the stress hormone cortisol can also rise when blood glucose levels are not well controlled. Remember, cortisol provides the body with protein for energy production (gluconeogenesis) by converting amino acids into usable carbohydrates (glucose) in the liver. Movement or exercise can help relieve physical and emotional stress, help with blood glucose control, and reduce levels of cortisol. Levels of cortisol can increase when blood glucose is not well controlled, which can cause even more resistance to insulin and greater challenges in getting blood glucose into a more normal range.[7]

One simple way to deal with stress is to move more. The way of wisdom teaches us to *"think about the ant! Consider its ways and be wise!"* (Proverbs 6:6) One characteristic of ants is that they keep moving. It is rare to see an ant just sitting.

There is a story about Tamerlane, an emperor who lived in the fourteenth century, and his army, which had been scattered by the enemy that relates to this. He was forced to hide in a deserted stable, while the enemy scoured the countryside. Later Tamerlane said, "I was forced to take shelter...where I sat alone many hours. Desiring to divert my mind from my hopeless condition, I fixed my eyes on an ant that was carrying a grain of corn larger than itself up a high wall. I numbered the efforts it made to accomplish this object. I counted that the ant dropped the grain sixty-nine times to the ground; but the insect persevered, and the seventieth time it reached the top. This sight gave me courage at the moment, and I never forgot the lesson." Yes, there is power in persistence; and for diabetes management, there is also power in persisting each day in movement.

Several benefits result when we are on the move. It provides a physical means to improve one's mood, helping a person face the stresses of life. Exercise actually stimulates the brain to release hormones called *endorphins*. Endorphins help with a more positive mood and also relieve the sensations of pain. Levels of serotonin are also increased, which help prevent depression.[8] Movement will be discussed in greater detail in chapter 11.

Blood Glucose Control: In chapter 2 we examined ways to better utilize glucose meters and where blood glucose levels should be. Did you know, however, that research done with those having Type 1 diabetes indicates that elevated levels of glucose contribute to a greater risk of depression? Researchers at the Joslin Diabetes Center discovered a link between high levels of glutamate and symptoms of depression. Glutamate is a neurotransmitter in the brain and is produced by glucose. Increased levels of glutamate were found in the area of the brain that is associated with both higher-level thinking and regulation of emotions. Another link that was found with the higher levels of glutamate was poor blood glucose control.[9] So not only does poor glucose control contribute to higher levels of cortisol, a stress hormone, it also contributes to higher levels of glutamate, which contributes to depression.

The 3 + 4 Plan: A third way (besides movement and better glucose control) to counter the physical effects of stress is to use the 3 + 4 plan. Three light meals and four healthy snacks two or three hours apart, spread throughout the day, equals better health. A study reported in the New England Journal of Medicine assigned fourteen men of average weight to two groups. Each group ate the same number of calories per day, in the same proportions of protein, carbohydrate, and fat. One group, however, only ate three large meals a day, whereas the other group ate seven light meals per day.

What were the results? Blood cholesterol levels fell by 15 percent. Cortisol, which is the stress related hormone (which can cause a resistance to insulin as well as requiring more insulin because of the release of converted amino acids to carbohydrate), dropped by 17 percent. The amount of insulin needed was also reduced by 28 percent. So instead of trying to eat just three times a day, eat three light meals and four healthy snacks two or three hours apart during the day.[10]

What about Snacks?

What are some more benefits of snacking? Snacking helps prevent overeating at meals, and it provides a constant source of nutritional fuel. Snacks help the body burn more calories, rather than storing them, by keeping the metabolic rate up. The body also gets a regular supply of fuel, which can help prevent low blood glucose levels when using insulin or sulfonylureas like Glipizide, Glimeperide, and Glyburide.[11]

What are some good snacks to eat? Fresh fruits, like a small apple, a cup or four ounces of cherries, half of a grapefruit, twelve grapes, an orange, a peach, or a pear could be used for snacks that do not drive up your blood sugars. They are all low–glycemic index carbohydrates, which do not spike up blood sugars. Raw vegetables also make good snacks. Eat them with a lower-fat dip or with different flavored mustards. Deli meat wrapped in lettuce leaves, low-fat cottage cheese and fruit, a boiled egg, or smoked salmon or tuna on whole grain crackers would all be good options for snacks as well. Portion control is essential for most of these snacks, however.

Gratitude: Another way the stress hormone cortisol was reduced was through a daily fifteen-minute practice of gratitude. After a month of doing this, a research group had an increase in a hormone called DHEA (dehydroepiandrosterone, which reflects physiological relaxation) and a reduction in cortisol. The research was done by the HeartMath organization.

The way the participants in the study practiced developing appreciation was by doing the following: They would focus on their hearts and even put their hands on their hearts. They were to sit calmly, breathing slowly, and focus on a genuine feeling of appreciation for someone or something positive in their lives. One person who had suffered two heart attacks and had quadruple bypass surgery started meditating for stress reduction by developing skills of highlighting appreciation, gratitude, and compassion in his life. This contributed to better levels of health and well-being.[12]

Remember, the way of wisdom states, *"Peace of mind means a healthy body, but jealousy will rot your bones"* (Proverbs 14:30). In summary, four ways to effectively cope with the negative effects of stress are to move more; keep better track of blood glucose levels, bringing them closer to normal (154 average or less); eat a light meal or snack about every two hours; and keep a gratitude dairy.

Also, in tense situations, use the wisdom principles of overlooking (not dwelling on) insults and offenses; focusing on good things; being patient; thinking before speaking; and using gentle words, not harsh words, when interacting with an upset person. *"Fools quickly show that they are upset, but the wise ignore insults"* (Proverbs 12:16). *"Whoever would foster love covers over an offense, but whoever repeats the matter separates close friends"* (Proverbs 17:9). *"Whoever looks for good will find kindness, but whoever looks for evil will find trouble"* (Proverbs 11:27). *"Patient people have great understanding, but people with quick tempers show their foolishness"* (Proverbs 14:29). *"A person's wisdom yields patience; it is to one's glory to overlook an offense"* (Proverbs 19:11). *"Good people think before they answer. Evil people have a quick reply, but it causes trouble"* (Proverbs 15:28). *"A gentle answer turns away wrath, but a harsh word stirs up anger"* (Proverbs 15:1). Finally, remember to keep this statement in mind: *"If you are wise, your wisdom will reward you"* (Proverbs 9:12).

1. Joseph P. Napora, PhD, *Stress-Free Diabetes: Your Guide to Health and Happiness* (Alexandria, Virginia: American Diabetes Association, 2010), 1–2.

2. Napora, 13–14.

3. Christine A. Maglione-Garves, Len Kravitz, PhD, and Suzanne Schneider, PhD, Cortisol Connection: Tips on Managing Stress and Weight http://www.unm.edu/~lkravitz/Article%20folder/stresscortisol.html (Accessed July 16, 2012)

4. S. I. McMillen, MD, and David E. Stern, MD, *None of These Diseases: The Bible's Health Secrets for the 21st Century* (Grand Rapids, MI: Fleming H. Revell, 2000), 209–10.

5. Gary Arsham, MD, and Ernest Lowe, Diabetes: A Guide to Living Well (Alexandria, Virginia: American Diabetes Association, 2004), 183-184.

6. Robert K. Cooper, PhD, Flip the Switch Lose the Weight: Proven Strategies to Fuel Your Metabolism & Burn Fat 24 Hours a Day (New York: Rodale Inc., 2005), 132-134.

7. Sheri R. Colberg, PhD, *The 7 Step Diabetes Fitness Plan: Living Well and Being Fit with Diabetes, No Matter Your Weight* (New York: Marlowe & Company, 2006), 153–54.

8. Richard Jackson, MD, and Amy Tenderich, *Know Your Numbers, Outlive Your Diabetes: Five Essential Health Factors You Can Master to Enjoy a Long and Healthy Life* (New York: Marlowe & Company, 2007), 104.

9. John Zrebiac, LICSW, and Gail Musen, PhD, Emotions & Blood-Sugar Levels: How Diabetes Can Affect Your Mood http://blog.joslin.org/2011/02/emotions-blood-sugar-levels-how-diabetes-can-affect-your-mood/ (Accessed July 16, 2012)

10. Robert K. Cooper, PhD, *Flip the Switch Lose the Weight: Proven Strategies to Fuel Your Metabolism & Burn Fat 24 Hours a Day* (New York: Rodale Inc., 2005), 204.

11. Karen Hanson Chalmers, RD, CDE, and Amy Peterson Campbell, RD, CDE, *16 Myths of a Diabetic Diet* (Alexandria, Virginia: American Diabetes Association, 2nd Edition, 2007), 170.

12. Robert A. Emmons, *Thanks: How Practicing Gratitude Can Make You Happier* (New York: Houghton Mifflin Company, 2007), 70, 73.

Chapter 9

Timing Is (Almost) Everything, Recording How You Are Doing, and Drinking Water

T iming
R ecord Keeping
I ce Water
U seful Satiety (Feel Full) Strategies
M ovement
P ortion Control
H ealthy Wisdom Principles
We'll examine each of these concepts in the next four chapters.

Timing Is (Almost) Everything

You've probably heard sayings about the importance of time like, "He was at the right place at the right time," or "Her timing was perfect." Is timing everything? Are you just waiting for energy and well-being to happen at the appropriate time? The following illustration shows the importance of timing.

While on a road trip, an elderly couple stopped at a roadside restaurant for lunch. After finishing their meal, they left the restaurant and resumed their trip. When leaving, the wife unknowingly left her glasses on the table, and she didn't miss them until after they had been driving about twenty minutes. By then, to add to the aggravation, they had to travel several miles before they could find a place to turn around to make their way back to retrieve her glasses.

All the way back, the elderly husband became the classic grouchy old man. He griped and complained during the entire trip back. The more he grumbled at her, the more agitated he became. He just wouldn't let up one minute. Finally, to her relief, they arrived at the restaurant. And, as the woman got out of the car and hurried inside to retrieve her glasses, the old geezer yelled to her, "While you're in there, you might as well get my hat and credit card." There was very little patience or kindness being displayed by this grouchy old husband! We all have to admit, however, his timing was perfect for retrieving his hat and credit card!

Of course, that little story dramatically demonstrates the importance of timing in relationships, but there is also the importance of timing in diabetes management. Timing issues can't be put off until tomorrow. One customer went into a furniture store and saw an old, faded sign that said, "Tomorrow we will give away everything in the store." At first the customer became excited until he realized tomorrow would never come. The sign had kept saying the same thing every day for years since it was now faded. Again, remember that the way of wisdom teaches principles that are for our health and well-being— *"they are life to those who find them and health to one's whole body"* (Proverbs 4:22).

Wisdom's way teaches the following on the importance of timing: *"Anyone who refuses to work doesn't plow in the right season. When he looks for a crop at harvest time, he doesn't find it"* (Proverbs 20:4). *"Finish your outdoor work. Get your fields ready. After that, build your house"* (Proverbs 24:27). *"A person finds joy in giving an apt reply—and how good is a timely word!"* (Proverbs 15:23). *"It is not good to have zeal without knowledge, nor to be hasty and miss the way"* (Proverbs 19:2).

It has been said, "Diabetes is like being expected to play the piano with one hand while juggling items with another hand, all while balancing with deftness and dexterity on a tightrope." Why is that? It's because we need to keep our blood sugars as close to normal as possible, which involves creating a meal plan with appropriate amounts and types of food, exercise, medication(s), and stress management. Add to that the importance of coordinating all those variables of management by applying their use at just the right times.

Weight control is a timing issue and is important for people with diabetes, because it relates to the sensitivity of insulin, especially with people with Type 2 diabetes. When one eats, as well as how quickly one eats, can influence weight control. It takes about twenty minutes before a person has that "feel full" feeling when eating. The timing of medications and of insulin must be considered for their most efficient use. Getting into a routine has to do with timing and will influence blood glucose management. The timing of metabolizing certain kinds of foods (like fatty foods) must be considered, as well as the timing of checking blood glucose levels.

Just recently I thought I had everything under control. I had an elevated blood sugar one morning and took a corrective dose of insulin. We were going to eat with family at a restaurant, but before going, I checked my blood sugar. My blood glucose level was on its way down. I thought by the time we would be served our food, I would be fine. Then something that shouldn't have been a surprise happened—we had to wait to be seated. I didn't even bother to bring my kit with me, which has my glucose meter. By the time we were finally seated, my blood sugar was coming down—way down! I became incoherent. My wife had to order for me and insisted I take some Smarties™! In this situation, timing is everything, isn't it? At least I had some Smarties™ and cooperated in taking them.

Weight Control

Have you ever seen sumo wrestlers? Their goal is to gain more weight, and they do so by gaining that weight in the waist. What is their secret to gaining weight? Their routine is to skip breakfast, exercise on an empty stomach, take a nap after eating, eat late in the day, and eat with others. After hearing about their routine, it would be easy to think that many people are in training to become sumo wrestlers, because that routine seems to be the American way.[1]

By skipping breakfast after a night of sleep, their metabolic rates can be kept lower. Then, by exercising on an empty stomach, they can better keep their bodies on a conservation mode to conserve energy rather than expend it. After exercising and eating a meal, they then take about a four-hour nap, which is another sumo secret for gaining weight. Another secret is to then eat late in the day. Going to bed with full stomachs means that their body's response is to store the excess fuel in fat cells. Another important factor is that they eat late with others.

Weight Control and Eating with Others

Research reported by Dr. Wansink indicates that there is power in norms—that is, what the average consumption of food is among a large group of people. The average amount others eat influences the appropriate amount that you think you should eat. The pace at which they eat can also be a factor on weight control. If you sit next to slow eaters, they can influence the pace at which you eat as well, which can result in eating less. On the other hand, sitting next to those who are speed eaters—who seem to have grown up in a family of twelve, where everyone was grappling for a morsel of food—will lead to more consumption. So, slow down with your fork. The slower pace allows satiety—the "I'm Full" signal—to kick in, which takes about twenty minutes.[2]

According to some researchers, one reason the French have a lower rate of heart disease is that they eat their main meal earlier in the day. This gives more time for physical activity after the meal. In fact, most French families consume 57 percent of their food for the day by 2:00 p.m. In contrast, Americans eat only 38 percent of their daily food by that time.

Also, a University of Minnesota study revealed that those who ate most of their calories earlier in the day lost 2.3 pounds per week on average. Those who ate most of their calories later in the day gained weight.[3] Timing is almost everything relative to when you consume most of your food. A good goal is to eat your main meal at noontime, rather than later in the day, like after 6:00 p.m.

Not only will eating late make it easier to gain weight, it also makes it more difficult to maintain blood sugar control. When you eat late, you have less time to exercise and burn the calories.

Remember to always eat your breakfast...and dinner and supper. (3 + 4 = SUCCESS—three light meals and four healthy snacks two to three hours apart, spread throughout the day.) Refer to chapter 8 for more information on the 3 + 4 eating plan.

Insulin Timing

Timing is almost everything when using insulin. Let me give you an example of what can happen with the timing of insulin and eating fatty foods. The length of time the insulin is active runs out before the fatty foods can be metabolized. Not keeping this in mind can happen to anyone, including people I know who have been injecting insulin with a syringe and needle for more than forty years and then using an insulin pump another ten.

There are two major types of insulin, short-acting and long-acting. In people without diabetes, insulin is released throughout the day for the basal metabolic rate, or BMR; likewise, a person with Type 1 diabetes also needs insulin throughout the day. The BMR is the amount of energy needed to support the work of the heart, brain, lungs, and other organs at rest, with no physical activity.[4]

Long-acting insulins like Lantus (glargine) and Levemir (determir) are used for the basal dose and are usually injected either once or twice a day. Rapid-acting insulins like Novolog, Apidra, and Humalog are used for meal coverage, the bolus, and take about twenty minutes to become active and last about four hours. When eating a meal, it's good to keep this in mind and take the insulin twenty minutes before eating, not after eating.[5]

What happens if a person takes the insulin after eating or doesn't take the appropriate amount? A high blood sugar reading is the result. To determine the proper amounts of insulin to be used, many use the 500 and 1500 rules. A person takes the TDD (total daily dosage) and divides 500 by that number. This gives the carb ratio, that is, how many grams of carbohydrate are covered by one unit of insulin.[6] If a person's TDD is 40, 500 would be divided by 40, giving a carb insulin ratio of about 12 grams of carbohydrate for every unit of insulin. A person can determine if the amount was accurate for a meal by checking the blood glucose level two hours **after starting to eat.**

Suppose a person checks the blood glucose level four hours after eating and discovers a count of 250. The target goal is 100, which means the number is 150 above the goal. The 1500 rule is then used for the correction. 1500 is divided by the TDD, which in this example is 40. From that ratio, each unit will lower the blood glucose by about 38 points. So 150 divided by 38 would mean the person should take about four units. Again, the timing is important, and it will take about four hours to bring the blood glucose to the target, because that is how long a rapid-acting insulin will last.

Keep in mind, these are only general rules and do not work perfectly and they are more accurate for people with Type 1 diabetes than those having Type 2 diabetes. If a person's blood glucose is 164, after having taken a correction dosage about three hours earlier, then there would be about one hour of rapid-acting insulin still on board, or 25 percent of the dosage. The person then goes to a restaurant with his family but ends up having to wait longer than expected to be seated and served. What can happen? Again, the timing is important, and the blood glucose could drop faster than expected. The person could then have a low blood sugar episode (hypoglycemia) and become so confused and disoriented that he can't even order his food. Of course, this is my own example, which I mentioned earlier in the chapter.

Do fatty foods increase blood glucose?

Someone says, "Your blood glucose is affected by sugar and carbs, so avoid them. Don't worry about other types of food!" However, wisdom's way says, *"The mind of a person with understanding gets knowledge; the wise person listens to learn more"* (Proverbs 18:15).

I've heard of some people eating fettuccine Alfredo with garlic bread and then finishing the meal with a dessert of Tiramisu. Two hours after starting to eat this meal, a blood glucose check is done and it is right on target with 129. But when the blood glucose is checked five hours after starting the meal, a number of 282 is discovered. The person thought the proper count of carbohydrates and the appropriate amount of rapid acting insulin was taken. By the way, in some restaurants the carbohydrate count would be a whopping 65 grams of carbohydrate for the fettuccine Alfredo and another 46 grams of carb for the Tiramisu, not even counting the bread.

Fettuccine Alfredo, garlic bread, Tiramisu, and pizza are a mixture of what kinds of food? They are a mixture of carbohydrates and fat. Fettuccine Alfredo is a dish consisting of fettuccine (pasta cut in flat narrow strips) with butter, Parmesan cheese, cream, and seasonings. Only a small portion of the fat molecule known as the *glycerol backbone* can be used as glucose. If fat doesn't directly raise blood glucose, what is it doing? Fat on the body used to be considered as just dead weight that people had to cart around all day long. Now it is known that losing visceral abdominal fat is very important. It is this fat that increases insulin resistance and glucose intolerance, lowers HDL-cholesterol, elevates triglycerides, and contributes to hypertension.[7]

Is fatty food just the shy, harmless guy sitting on the back row?

When fatty foods are eaten, they have a powerful metabolic punch. Free fatty acids (FFAs) in the blood increase with high–saturated fat meals. What does that do? Insulin resistance also increases with high–saturated fat meals. That resistance means that it will take more insulin to break through the insulin resistance barrier to move the glucose from the bloodstream into the cells.

Fat also changes the timing of the rise in blood glucose after a meal, because fat takes up to six hours to move through the gastrointestinal tract. How long does rapid-acting insulin such as Novolog, Humalog, or Apidra stay active? They stay active for about four hours. When you eat a high-fat meal, the insulin is done working before a significant amount of glucose reaches the blood. The action of the insulin runs out before the rest of the glucose makes an appearance because of the slowing process of fat.

The following is the American Heart Association's guidelines for fat consumption: Limit total fat intake to less than 25–35 percent of your total calories each day, and limit saturated fat intake to less than 7 percent of total daily calories. This means that a 2000-calorie meal plan could include 140 calories from saturated fat, or 16 grams. It is also best to not eat those 16 grams all in one sitting.

Reduce consumption of saturated fats like red meat and dairy products. Think chicken, turkey, and low-fat or skim milk. Monounsaturated fats like olives, avocados, cashews, almonds, peanuts, and olive and peanut oil actually lower LDL ("bad") cholesterol and insulin resistance and raise HDL. Polyunsaturated fats are found in salmon, herring, tuna, cod, pumpkin, and sunflower seeds and oil, as well as in corn oil. They also lower LDL cholesterol and triglyceride levels.[8]

What should we do?

Avoid meals containing 40 or more grams of fat, especially if the fat is saturated. Alter the amount and timing of your insulin if you eat high-fat meals, taking an additional smaller dose later. For people with Type 2 diabetes taking oral medications, as well as those on insulin, doing some type of physical activity—for example, walking after a high-fat meal—can help control blood glucose.[9]

Someone might say, "I love my Fettuccine Alfredo, garlic bread, Tiramisu, pizza, chocolate candy, French fries, and fried chicken too much to give up!" Another person, however, who is trying to follow the way of wisdom, remembers that *"The wise see danger ahead and avoid it, but fools keep going and get into trouble"* (Proverbs 22:3).

Record Keeping—Know the Condition of Your Health and Life, and Keep a Daily Personal Health Inventory

"Keep good records of your blood sugars, food, and movement levels" is the advice given to a person who's been recently diagnosed with diabetes. That person reacts by saying, "You've got to be kidding! I've never done anything like that before. It sounds like more trouble than it's worth." In contrast, wisdom's way teaches one to keep a personal inventory of health. Proverbs 27:23 puts the principle this way: *"Be sure you know the condition of your flocks, give careful attention to your herds."* Of course, I know few people who have flocks or herds, but the principle is to know the condition of what you have. It applies to knowing our own personal health inventory, that is, the things we are doing to be healthy. It is important to know where your blood sugar level is. What is just as important is to keep a record of what you're eating, how many steps you are taking, and what the resulting blood sugar levels are. Keeping a health record gives you the opportunity to make educated changes or adjustments in your regimen! *"The simple believe anything, but the prudent give thought to their steps"* (Proverbs 14:15).

If your doctor's office calls to let you know your last A1c test result, and the caller tells you that the doctor says it looks fine, should that be good enough? (The A1c test gives the average blood glucose for a three-month period. For more information on the A1c, read chapter 2.) Dr. Richard Jackson of the Joslin Diabetes Center says, "Imagine going up to a bank teller and asking how much money you have in your account. The teller looks up your records and tells you, 'Not to worry, you are fine.'"[10] Would you be satisfied with that answer? Wouldn't you want to know exactly what you have? That would certainly help with the financial decisions you need to make, wouldn't it? What if you didn't look at your savings account for a month and then discovered that someone had gotten access to your bank account and spent three thousand dollars? We need to keep track of our own physical condition, too, knowing the average blood glucose and A1c numbers as well as blood pressure and cholesterol levels. In other words, keep your own daily records!

Surveys reveal that most people are amazingly unaware of how much they eat in the evening. In fact, most people have difficulty in keeping track of their food consumption. "The first, and perhaps the most important, lifestyle behavior is to keep records," says Kelly D. Brownell, PhD, codirector of the Eating and Weight Disorders Clinic at Yale University. Those who most accurately recorded their food consumption lost the most weight, according to the *Journal of the American Dietetic Association*.[11]

You can keep records by putting the amounts you eat in a daily food journal, along with blood sugar readings and a daily gratitude list. By keeping records, you will be able to answer the following questions: Do you always have a snack while watching TV? Is a second or third helping for a meal automatic? Do you tend to order the bigger meal, because it is a better deal? Do you eat before bed? Do you skip breakfast and overeat later in the day? Write down everything you eat, immediately after you eat, including the amounts. *"When you sit down to eat with a ruler, observe carefully what is before you"* (Proverbs 23:1).

If you only check your blood glucose two or three times a day, you can vary the times you check. Don't always check at the same time each day, except when you get up in the morning. Use the "pairs" method—that is, take blocks of time like lunchtime, checking your blood glucose before eating and two hours after starting to eat. By doing this, the effect of what you eat will be seen on blood glucose. Do this for three days in a row to see if adjustments need to be made on the selection of foods and then move on to supper time. By recording your results, patterns will become apparent. If there is a pattern of highs, you will know changes need to be made in either meal planning, movement (exercise) times, or medication.[12]

You can take the guesswork out of management, because you will have records that will show you what you need to know. Not only do I keep track of what I eat, the amount of movement (numbers of steps per day), and blood glucose readings, but I also include the five things for which I am thankful in my journal.

Ice Water—"Like cold water to a weary soul is good news from a distant land" (Proverbs 25:25).

"You want me to drink water? It's too boring!" If it is too boring, add a sugar-free flavoring, which you can find next to the Kool-Aid™ in the grocery store! Dehydration makes a person feel fatigued. Remember, when reading the proverb above, the statement that is made of God's wisdom teachings in Proverbs 4:22 - *"They are life to those who find them and health to one's whole body."* The basic meaning of the word *proverb* is *represent, compare,* or *be like.* Proverbs are pictures of reality. What better way to picture the gratifying, exuberant effect that good news has on a person than with the picture of the satisfaction cold water gives a really thirsty person? *"Like cold water to a weary soul is good news from a distant land"* (Proverbs 25:25).

Proverbs have more than one dimension, and the meaning here is not just about good news. In other words, the consequence of good news is pictured with the wonderful feeling that cold water gives to a thirsty person. And guess what? Cold water is good for our health.

A hungry feeling between meals may actually be a symptom of thirst. When you feel hungry, instead of eating something, try drinking a glass of water. Wait ten minutes and then see how you feel.

Dr. Willett of Harvard Medical School suggests drinking sixty-four ounces of water a day for a person on a 2,000-calorie meal plan.[13] Others have suggested drinking half an ounce for every pound you weigh and an ounce for every minute you exercise to keep hydrated. Why is this so important for those with diabetes? Wisdom's way teaches that *"The mind of a person with understanding gets knowledge; the wise person listens to learn more"* (Proverbs 18:15).

In a nine-year study of 3,615 men and women who had normal blood sugar at the beginning of the study, research was conducted to see if staying hydrated lowers the risk of high blood sugars. French researchers indicated that drinking at least thirty-two ounces of water per day could reduce the chances of developing elevated blood sugar problems. Those who drank more than thirty-two ounces of water per day were 21 percent less likely to develop high blood sugar than those who drank sixteen ounces or less daily. The analysis also took into account other factors that can affect the risk of elevated blood sugar, to get an accurate picture of the significance of water consumption.[14]

"Studies have shown that being just half a liter dehydrated can increase your cortisol levels," says Amanda Carlson, RD, director of performance nutrition at Athletes' Performance, a trainer of world-class athletes. "Cortisol is one of those stress hormones. Staying in a good hydrated status can keep your stress levels down. When you don't give your body the fluids it needs, you're putting stress on it, and it's going to respond to that," says Amanda Carlson.[15] Two stress hormones, cortisol and epinephrine, are released by the brain when under stress. These two hormones can cause a resistance to the available insulin, causing an elevation in blood sugar levels and a greater need for available insulin.

A simple way to relax and contribute to better blood sugar control is to make it a point to drink a glass of water after a stress-filled event. Better yet, make it a habit to drink small amounts of water throughout the day. Six glasses all at once isn't good for you! *"The wisdom of the prudent is to give thought to their ways"* (Proverbs 14:8).

1. Robert K. Cooper, PhD, *Flip the Switch Lose the Weight: Proven Strategies to Fuel Your Metabolism & Burn Fat 24 Hours a Day* (New York: Rodale Inc., 2005), 98.

2. Brian Wansink, PhD, *Mindless Eating: Why We Eat More Than We Think* (New York: Bantam Dell, 2006), 99.

3. Cooper, 142–44.

4. Boris Draznin, MD, *Living With Diabetes: Dr. Draznin's Plan for Better Health* (New York: Oxford University Press, Inc., 2008), 29.

5. Richard Beaser, MD, ed., *Joslin Diabetes Deskbook: A Guide for Primary Care Providers* (Boston: Joslin Diabetes Center, 2010), 270.

6. Beaser, 126–27.

7. Beaser, 82.

8. Lucy Beale, RD, CDE, and Joan Clark, RD, CDE, *Glycemic Index Weight Loss: Easy-to-Follow Diet Plans That Keep Your Weight Low and Metabolism High* (New York: Penguin Group, 2005), 116–18.

9. Joslin Communications, Why Does Fat Increase Blood Glucose? http://blog.joslin.org/2011/09/why-does-fat-increase-blood-glucose/#.TqadrlVmud4.email (Accessed July 16, 2012)

10. Steven V. Edelman, MD, *Taking Control of Your Diabetes* (West Islip, New York: Professional Communications, Inc., 2007), 52.

11. Cooper, 144.

12. Beaser, 63.

13. Walter Willett, MD, *Eat, Drink, and Weigh Less: A Flexible and Delicious Way to Shrink your Waist Without Going Hungry* (New York: Tante Malka, Inc., 2006), 67.

14. Charlene Laino, Drinking Water May Cut Risk of High Blood Sugar http://diabetes.webmd.com/news/20110630/drinking-water-may-cut-risk-of-high-blood-sugar (Accessed July 3, 2012)

15. Gina Shaw, "Water and Stress Reduction: Sipping Stress Away" http://www.webmd.com/diet/features/water-stress-reduction (Accessed July 3, 2012)

Chapter 10

Eating More, Feeling Full, and Losing Weight

What is the best approach to losing weight? Is getting in a hurry to lose weight the best approach? Does a patient approach carry a lot of wait—or weight? Is the gradual approach the most effective? How can food cravings be managed, especially when trying to lose weight? Are there certain kinds of foods that will best satisfy those cravings and keep those who are patient on the right track with blood sugar levels? What other obstacles are there? What about a lack of support and encouragement from others, or ignorance about the "how to's" of meal planning? How can eating salads help? What wisdom guidelines reinforce the best eating? Let's examine the answers.

Many with Type 2 diabetes can reduce or completely eliminate oral medications by just losing weight, because there is improved sensitivity to insulin. Eighty-five percent of people with diabetes are overweight when diagnosed. A loss of just 5 to 7 percent, which for many people is just ten to twenty pounds, will cause the body's sensitivity to insulin to improve remarkably.

A good way to start losing weight is to first determine how much you can eat per day without gaining weight. A good guideline to follow is to multiply your current weight by eleven. If you weigh about 230 pounds, multiply that number by eleven to get the total number of calories you can eat without gaining weight, which in this case would be about 2,500 calories. You can think of this as your calorie ceiling, assuming your activity level is about the same each day.

Second, to lose fifteen pounds, which would be about 7 percent of your weight if you weigh 230 pounds, subtract 500 hundred calories per day to lose a pound per week. This is a general guideline that works for most people.[1] This method, along with movement, which we'll examine in the next chapter, will reduce a certain kind of fat known as *visceral fat*. Why is losing visceral abdominal fat so important? It's important because this kind of fat increases insulin resistance and glucose intolerance (for example, elevated blood glucose levels after eating), lowers HDL-cholesterol (the good cholesterol), elevates triglycerides, and contributes to hypertension.[2]

How to Turn Obstacles into Stepping Stones for a More Healthy Future

---

There are many barriers that have to be overcome to lose weight, including the following:

People Obstacles: Friends are there to help you gain weight, but where are they when you're trying to lose weight? There is a cartoon that shows two overweight ladies coming out of a Baskin-Robbins ice cream shop. One says, "Don't worry about your dietician finding out, Allison. What happens in Baskin-Robbins stays in Baskin-Robbins." Is that friend really being helpful? When you cheat on your meal plan or exercise, you are only cheating yourself. It doesn't affect your doctor, dietician, or friend. Some people feel embarrassed when a friend or relative starts trying to lose weight, because they feel guilty about not doing so themselves. They might try to convince you to stop making those changes. Some people could be described as basement people—they try to drag you back down to the old lifestyle. On the other hand, other people could be described as balcony people, as they are trying to lift you up and encourage your efforts for healthy living. Find people who will encourage you, not discourage you! *"Spend time with the wise and you will become wise, but the friends of fools will suffer"* (Proverbs 13:20).

Meal Planning Obstacle: Maybe you're not sure how to follow a meal plan. Someone said, "My doctor told me about the importance of a healthy meal plan, which—as best as I can tell—means I'm only allowed to eat birdseed all day." A healthy meal plan is not boring and mundane! Proper, tasty meal planning involves eating more but with less calories, and birdseed is not on the menu.

Getting in a Big Hurry Obstacle: Being in a big hurry to lose weight is a common mistake. It is estimated that 95 percent of people who go on deprivation diets end up gaining back all the weight they lost. The body's metabolism furnace, its conservation switch, turns on when too little food is eaten for the body's needs. It is like an SOS goes out, telling the body to store fat, because the famine is coming. Eat too little, and the body will go into conservation mode, making it even harder to burn off the pounds. Some people can do it; however, once the goal is reached, they quickly gain back what they lost. No constructive habits were formed in the process. Horace Mann said, "Habits are like a cable. We weave a strand of it every day, and soon it cannot be broken." That is, they are very hard to break, which is good when the habits help instead of hurt.[3]

The patient approach is what is needed. It's been said that the shortest period of time in America is when the light turns green and you hear the first horn honk. If you don't leave immediately, someone behind you is going to quickly honk their horn! We live in a microwave, fast-food-mentality society. Wisdom's way teaches, *"Those who are patient have great understanding, but the quick-tempered display folly,"* and *"It is not good to have zeal without knowledge, nor to be hasty and miss the way"* (Proverbs 14:29, 19:2).

Patience Carries a Lot of Wait, But It Works: Counting the Small Stuff

---

Jean says, "I have FORTY pounds to lose! I have tried every diet there is. I am not going to waste my time on all this small stuff!" Let's consider the following humorous story and then read the example of Cindy to get a better perspective on the power of doing little things. They can add up and make a positive impact!

The story is told of a country lad who was hired for a sales job at a city department store. It was one of those massive stores that has every department imaginable. In fact, it was the biggest store in the world—you could get anything there. The boss said, "You can start tomorrow, Friday morning, and I'll come and see you when we close."

When the boss looked up the young man the next day at closing time, he saw him shaking hands with a beaming customer. After they parted, he walked over and asked, "Well, that looked good! How many sales did you make today?"

"That was the only one," said the young salesman.

"Only one!" exclaimed the boss. "Most of my staff makes twenty or thirty sales a day. You'll have to do better than that! Well, how much was the sale worth?"

"$227,340 and change," said the young man.

The boss stood speechless for a moment, blinking a few times. "How did you manage to do that?"

"Well, when he came in this morning, I sold him a small fish hook. Then, I sold him a medium hook, and then a really large hook. Then I sold him a small fishing line, a medium one, and then a big one. I then sold him a spear gun, a wetsuit, scuba gear, nets, and coolers. I asked him where he was going fishing, and he said down the coast. We decided he would probably need a new boat, so I took him down to the boat department and sold him that twenty-foot schooner with the twin engines. Then, he said that his Volkswagen probably wouldn't be able to pull it, so I took him to the truck department and sold him the new Deluxe Cruiser, with a winch, storage rack, rust proofing, and a built-in refrigerator. Oh, and floor mats."

The boss took two steps back and asked in astonishment, "You sold all that to a guy who came in for a fish hook?"

"No," answered the salesman. "He came in to buy a blanket."

"A blanket?"

"Yeah, an extra blanket for the couch. He just had a fight with his wife. I said to him, 'Well, your weekend is ruined, so you may as well go fishing....'" One thing leads to another! It works the same way for gaining weight. Calories add up and can easily lead to a gain of five pounds a year. All it takes is fifty extra calories a day that you don't utilize. Fifty calories is like two chocolate kisses. The good news is that when fifty calories is cut back each day, five pounds can also be lost in a year. Yes, one thing leads to another.

Cindy, a colleague of Dr. Wansink, lost twenty pounds after working at a new job for two years. How did she do it? The only deliberate change she made was to give up caffeine. She switched from coffee to herbal tea, but that didn't seem to answer anything. "Oh, yeah," she said, "and because I gave up caffeine, I also stopped drinking Coke." She had been drinking about six cans a week, which meant that she had cut back about 140 calories a day. That meant that she could have lost about fourteen pounds per year, and she actually lost about twenty pounds in two years.[4]

Keep Working Patiently on the Small Stuff, Because Life Has a Way of Accumulating

---

The wisdom way principle states that *"Whoever gathers money little by little makes it grow"* (Proverbs 13:11). There is truth in the saying "Inch by inch, life's a cinch; yard by yard, life is hard." Wisdom's way also teaches *"Those who are patient have great understanding"* (Proverbs 14:29). *"If you are wise, your wisdom will reward you"* (Proverbs 9:12). We'll be wise if we don't expect results instantly. We can patiently wait for good results by doing more movement and more eating of tasty, filling, and nutritious foods. By having the mind-set to patiently do things, gaining control little by little over weight and blood sugars, proper habits will be formed.

Choosing Foods That Are Less Concentrated in Calories

Many people think that certain kinds of foods, commonly called *comfort foods*, will fill them up, but instead they soon are craving more. Some of the most popular comfort foods—which people with diabetes shouldn't make a habit of eating anyway—are potato chips, ice cream, cookies, candy, and chocolate. The way of wisdom teaches us to continue to learn—*"Intelligent people are always open to new ideas. In fact, they look for them"* (Proverbs 18:15).

Did you know that a donut hole, which weighs only half an ounce, has fifty-two calories? However, 5.1 ounces of strawberries has only forty-six calories! Which one do you think will give you a more full feeling? Low-calorie density foods, which add more volume of food to your plate, but with fewer calories, are foods that give a "feel full feeling." A donut hole is a high-density calorie food because it has three grams of fat. On the other hand, the 5.1-ounce serving of strawberries has virtually no fat, but it has water and three grams of fiber.

The following quote from the Mayo Clinic has implications for our blood glucose control and weight. They say, "Choosing foods that are less concentrated with calories—meaning you get a larger portion size with a fewer number of calories—can help you lose weight and control your hunger."[5] The way of wisdom teaches, *"Be careful what you think, because your thoughts run your life"* (Proverbs 4:23). In this case, think *volume* of foods like vegetables, fruits, and lean meat. Eating more vegetables and fruits, which are mainly comprised of water with some fiber, will help provide a much longer full feeling than foods that have a high concentration of fat.

Foods are categorized by calorie density or high density, low density at the www.calorieking.com with asterisks. For example, strawberries are given four asterisks while the donut hole previously mentioned is given one asterisk. Foods with four asterisks would be the foods that are very low in calories per gram. The fewer asterisks a food has the greater number of calories it has per gram. Let's notice what wisdom's way teaches, as well as what we learn from research studies, on the benefits of low-calorie foods for health and well-being.

Are You a Meat and Potatoes Person, or Are You a Vegetables and Fruit Person?

Remember, these sayings or proverbs *"are the key to life for those who find them; they bring health to the whole body"* (Proverbs 4:22). Proverbs 18:20 teaches the importance of how people speak to one another. Sometimes emotional stress is heightened by the very words that are used with others. And stress has its effects on blood sugar levels, as we've previously examined. Some people vent their anger with words they later regret. The way of wisdom teaches, *"A gentle answer turns away wrath, but a harsh word stirs up anger"* (Proverbs 15:1). The basic meaning of Proverbs 18:20 is this: *"People will be rewarded for what they say; they will be rewarded by how they speak,"* or *"You will have to live with the consequences of everything you say."* A more literal translation of the original Hebrew to English says this: *"From the fruit of their mouths people's stomachs are filled; with the harvest of their lips they are satisfied."*

When I read the word *fruit*, it brings to mind a positive mind-set of what is tasty and nutritious. Most types of fruit have plenty of fiber and are slowly metabolized, not causing the blood sugar levels to spike up. We know the major teaching of the passage has to do with the consequences of what people say, but the principle would also apply to the consequences of what people eat.

It's interesting that the way of wisdom teaches, *"Be careful what you think, because your thoughts run your life"* (Proverbs 4:23). The picture being used for the good use of one's words is fruit. Fruit, in a good sense, is also used in the Bible to talk about the literal produce or fruit of trees (Genesis 1:12, Proverbs 27:18). In this case, a likeness or picture of something that is nutritious and beneficial to one's health is used. Fruit, a tasty, healthy food, is used to bring to our minds the healthy results or consequences of using the proper language with others.

Proverbs have more than one dimension. They are carefully crafted sayings of "compressed experience" from generations of wise people. They are rich with meaning, having more insights for living than what is obvious on the surface. Their purpose is to picture reality. The basic meaning of the word *proverb* is represent, compare, or be like.[6] Not only is the teaching of Proverbs 18:20 helpful for communicating in a rewarding way, but the very picture of fruit is, too. Let's look at what literal fruit in the stomach will do.

Feel Full on Less Calories: Research Studies

As previously mentioned, eating foods that make you feel full have a high percentage of water content. Notice the water content of the following foods: fruits and vegetables (80–95%), hot cereal (85%), low-fat fruit-flavored yogurt (75%), boiled egg (75%), and fish and seafood (60–85%). When we compare a popular junk food like potato chips, we discover it has only 2 percent water content.[7]

Researchers at Penn State University conducted a clinical trial for one year with seventy-one obese women age twenty-two to sixty. They wanted to determine if eating low-calorie, dense foods would facilitate the loss of weight as well as control hunger. They were assigned to one of two groups, each with different meal plan emphases. One was a meal plan with a reduced fat content and the other group also had a reduced fat content, plus they were to eat foods high in water content. Neither group was assigned a limit to the amount of calories they could eat each day. As people with diabetes, however, we do need to keep track of how many carbohydrates we eat, because carbs do affect blood glucose control.

Weight was lost by both groups of women. The group that added more low-density calorie foods, the water-rich foods, ate 25 percent more food by weight, not calories; felt less hungry; and lost more weight. After six months, those on the meal plan of reduced fat lost 14.7 pounds, whereas the other group lost 19.6 pounds. "We have now shown that choosing foods that are low in calorie density helps in losing weight, without the restrictive messages of other weight loss diets," explained Dr. Julia A. Ello-Martin.[8]

What Can We Learn from Daniel?

As a captive in Babylon during the reign of king Nebuchadnezzar (605–562 BC), Daniel and his three friends were being trained to be wise men in the royal courts. Their acclimation into the Babylonian culture included what they would eat and drink and was decided by the king. Daniel objected that the food would defile him spiritually, so he appealed to the officer to let them eat vegetables instead. The officer said, *"What would happen if he saw that you looked malnourished in comparison to the other young men your age?"* Daniel said to him, *"Please test your servants for ten days by providing us with some vegetables to eat and water to drink. Then compare our appearance with that of the young men who are eating the royal delicacies; deal with us in light of what you see"* (Daniel 1:10,12-13). What happened?

"So the guard agreed. He tested them for ten days. After the ten days they looked healthy and well fed. In fact, they looked better than any of the young men who ate the king's food" (Daniel 1:11–15). We've examined the importance of water and water-rich foods like fruits and vegetables for health and well-being. It worked 2,700 years ago, and it will still work today!

A Proverb about a Meal of Vegetables

Remember that the basic meaning of the word proverb is represent, compare or be like. Proverbs give pictures of life. Notice how the picture of love and hatred is contrasted and portrayed in the following Proverb: *"Better a meal of vegetables where there is love than a fattened calf with hatred"* (Proverbs 15:17). Most people find a meal of delicious steak very satisfying to the taste, but the taste is lost when eating the meal with those who are bitter, resentful and hateful toward you. Whereas, the picture of a meal with those you love is pictured with vegetables. And guess what? As we've been examining vegetables are good for us. Isn't it interesting that a subtle message of a meal with love is portrayed with vegetables, which are very beneficial to good health and not something that isn't beneficial?

Why Eating a Salad before the Main Course Can Make a Positive Difference

---

What would happen if you ate a salad before each meal? Would it affect the amount of calories you would eat for the entire meal? Forty-two women participated in a study conducted by the Department of Nutritional Sciences of Penn State University to research that very idea. Several lunch options were given for each lunch. The control condition was to not eat a salad before the main course of the meal, which was pasta. They were to eat as much pasta as they desired, and the amount of calories was measured.

Other lunch options were various sizes and energy densities of salads. The participants were required to eat the salads before the main course. The portion size of the salads used was either 150 grams or 300 grams of weight. The energy density of the salad was reduced by changing the amount and type of dressing and cheese. Obviously, the salad ended up being smaller when more dressing or cheese was used, bringing the weight to either 150 grams or 300 grams, but with less lettuce or vegetables. For example, the 150-gram salad came with three levels of total calories: fifty, one hundred, or two hundred calories. If it was the low-energy-density salad, it would be equal to about three cups of salad with a very light dressing. The 300-gram salad came with the same calculations (0.33, 0.67, or 1.33 kcal/g, or one hundred, two hundred, or four hundred total calories).[9]

According to this study, if you want to control weight or lose weight, eat a salad without high-calorie dressings or cheese before your main course at dinner or supper. When the low-energy-density salads were eaten—that, is the salads that pack more volume of food on the plate or in the bowl, but with fewer calories—less food was eaten during the main course of pasta. In other words, starting a meal with this type of salad enhances satiety or the feeling of being full and thus reduces the amount of calories eaten during the main course.

The study further determined that a salad for weight loss is an effective strategy when a large portion is eaten before meals. For the smaller salad of 150 grams, with a low-calorie dressing, 7 percent less was eaten for the main course; and for the 300-gram salad, it was 12 percent. A practical application of this is to take the pre-packaged salads (like iceberg) and make a salad with two servings, or three cups, which is thirty calories; and add a serving of low-calorie vinaigrette dressing, which is another thirty calories, for a grand total of sixty calories.

According to the research, if you use calorie-rich dressings like blue cheese, which has seventy-six calories and 8 grams of fat per serving, or Thousand Island dressing, which has sixty calories and almost 6 grams of fat, you will end up eating more for the main course. When two salads with the same number of calories were compared, it was found that meal intake was decreased when the large portion of the lower-energy-density salad was consumed; and meal intake was increased with the smaller portion of energy-dense salad. The message is to leave off the rich dressings! Use the low-calorie dressings, like vinaigrette, and have more salad!

What Are the Right Kinds of Sandwiches to Eat?

Several research studies at Penn State under the direction of Dr. Barbara Rolls have shown that volume of food trumps calories. We tend to eat the volume we want, not the calories we want. If a person feels full after eating a half-pound hamburger, what would happen if a quarter pound was used instead, along with plenty of lettuce, tomato, and onion added to make it appear to be the same size? Even though the quarter-pound hamburger had far fewer calories, those who ate it rated themselves as feeling just a full as they did with a half-pound hamburger.[10]

Of course, when it comes to eating sandwiches, a better choice would be meat with less saturated fat, like a six-inch turkey breast sandwich. It only has 280 calories, with 46 grams of carbohydrates, 5 grams of fiber, and only 3.5 grams of fat. When I get one of these sandwiches, I ask them to heap the lettuce and other vegetables on it, which makes the sandwich look (and be) bigger, but with just a few extra calories. Better yet, when having a sandwich wrap it with leaves of romaine lettuce instead of bread, which will really make a difference in blood sugar control. On the other hand, the quarter-pound hamburger has about 510 calories and 26 grams of fat. As we learned in chapter 9, this much fat can cause a delayed spike in your blood sugars several hours later.

Is There Any Evidence That Food Puffed Up with Air Is More Satisfying than Food That Is Denser?

Another research study was done with strawberry smoothies. They put the same ingredients in the blender but varied the time they were blended. The only difference was the air that got whipped into it.

Some smoothies only filled half a glass; others, with the longer duration of whipping, filled the glass. Would it make any difference in how satisfying and filling it would be?

When the half glass of smoothie was given to male college students compared to the full glass, there was a sharp contrast in the meals they ate thirty minutes later. Those who had the full glass ate 12 percent less, felt fuller, and didn't make up the calories later in the day. Dr. Rolls concludes that when you pump up the volume, "you see a bigger portion, and you get more sensory stimulation as you consume it." One way to put this into practice is to use air-popped popcorn and look for cereals that are flaky or puffed.[11]

"A wise man keeps himself under control"
(Proverbs 29:11).

These ideas of using foods that have more volume instead of calories are a smart way to practice self-control. The way of wisdom teaches self-control. *"Like a city whose walls are broken through is a person who lacks self-control"* (Proverbs 25:28). *"Better a patient man than a warrior, a man who controls his temper than one who takes a city"* (Proverbs 16:32). Self-control is needed in emotional interactions with others as well as when one eats. It's a wise, healthy defense habit for wellness. Mindless eating and mindlessly using words with others are not the kinds of habits that contribute to health and well-being. One adds weight, and the other adds stress to one's life—neither of which is helpful for self-management of diabetes.

The story is told of a principal of a small middle school, who had a problem with what a few of the older girls were doing with their lipstick. After applying it in the bathroom, they would then press their lips to the mirror and leave lip prints.

Before it got out of hand, he thought of a way to stop it. He gathered all the girls together who wore lipstick and told them he wanted to meet with them in the ladies' room at 2:00 p.m. They gathered at 2:00 p.m. and found the principal and the school custodian waiting for them.

The principal explained that it was becoming a problem for the custodian to clean the mirror every night. He said he felt the girls did not fully understand just how much of a problem it was, and he wanted them to witness firsthand just how hard it was to clean.

The custodian then demonstrated. He took a long-handled brush out of a box. He then dipped the brush in the nearest toilet, moved to the mirror and proceeded to remove the lipstick. That was the last time the girls ever pressed their lips to the mirror! It was disgusting.

We, too, can break bad habits and develop good eating habits for our own health and well-being. When it comes to diabetes, unhealthy eating habits lead to poor blood glucose control and then complications, which is something that no one desires. The most prevalent complication is neuropathy (nerve damage of the legs, feet, and arms). It affects as many as 75 percent of people with diabetes.[12] Remember, *"Those who get wisdom love their own lives; those who cherish understanding will soon prosper"* (Proverbs 19:8). These "feel full on more food, but with less calories" strategies will help achieve better blood sugar levels, weight control, and health. Let's use them!

1. Robert Buynak, MD, Dr. *Buynak's 1-2-3 Diabetes Diet: A Step-by-Step Approach to Weight Loss without Gimmicks or Risks* (Alexandria, Virginia: American Diabetes Association, 2006), 13, 85.

2. Richard Beaser, MD, ed., *Joslin Diabetes Deskbook: A Guide for Primary Care Providers* (Boston: Joslin Diabetes Center, 2010), 82.

3. Brian Wansink, PhD, *Mindless Eating: Why We Eat More than We Think* (New York: Bantam Dell, 2007), 25–27.

4. Wansink, 31.

5. Mayo Clinic Staff, Energy density and weight loss: Feel full on fewer calories http://www.mayoclinic.com/health/weight-loss/NU00195 (Accessed July 16, 2012)

6. Eldon Woodcock, *Proverbs: A Topical Study* (Grand Rapids: Zondervan Publishing House, 1988), 11.

7. Barbara Rolls, PhD, *The Volumetrics Eating Plan: Techniques and Recipes for Feeling Full on Fewer Calories* (New York: HarperCollins Publishers, 2005), 10.

8. Penn State (2007, June 8). Calorie Density Key To Losing Weight. ScienceDaily. http://www.sciencedaily.com/releases/2007/06/070608093819.htm (Accessed July 16, 2012)

9. Barbara Rolls, PhD, Salad and Satiety: Energy Density and Portion Size of a First-Course Salad Affect Energy Intake at Lunch, Department of Nutritional Sciences, The Pennsylvania State University, http://www.ncbi.nlm.nih.gov/pubmed/15389416 - October, 2004 (Accessed July 17, 2012)

10. Wansink, 44–45.

11. Barbara Rolls, PhD, *The Volumetrics Weight-Control Plan: Feel Full on Fewer Calories!* (New York: HarperTorchCollins, 2003), 20–21.

12. Marvin A. Levine, MD, ed. and Michael A. Pfeifer, MD, ed., *The Uncomplicated Guide to Diabetes Complications: What Every Person with Diabetes Needs to Know about Prevention, Treatment, and Self-Care for Complications of the Heart, Nerves, Feet, Eyes, Skin, Kidneys and More* (Alexandria, Virginia: American Diabetes Association, 2009), 157.

Chapter 11

Keeping on the Move

After World War II, a young lieutenant and his general got on a passenger train in London, or so the story goes. They were seated across from a grandmother and her beautiful granddaughter. A few minutes later, the train entered a tunnel. For about ten seconds, everyone was in the dark, and during that time they heard two things: a kiss and a slap!

Everyone assumed they knew what happened. The grandmother was thinking, "The audacity of that young soldier, but at least she had the nerve to slap him back!" In conversation before the kiss, the beautiful granddaughter was starting to like the lieutenant. She didn't really mind the kiss, but she was embarrassed that her grandmother had slapped him. The general was thinking, "Now, that's my lieutenant, but why did she have to slap me?" The young lieutenant was the only one who actually knew what happened. He saw the ten seconds of darkness as an opportunity to kiss the beautiful granddaughter and slap his general!

That is a cute little story, isn't it? As you read the story, it was easy to fall for the assumptions each of them was making. However, you may be wondering, what does this have to do with exercise and diabetes? Well, we, too, can make assumptions about what we need to do when it comes to exercise. When you think of exercise, what do you assume? Are you thinking workout, calisthenics, aerobics, exertion, running, jogging, power walking, or hour-long walks? And does the way of wisdom have anything to say about this?

"Go to the Ant, Consider Its Ways, and Be Wise"

"Go to the ant, you sluggard; consider its ways and be wise! It has no commander, no overseer or ruler, yet it stores its provisions in summer and gathers its food at harvest" (Proverbs 6:6–8). *"Ants are creatures of little strenght, yet they store up their food in the summer"* (Proverbs 30:25).

Just think of ants! What are some of their characteristics? They are fast and strong. Ants take the initiative. They don't let obstacles get in their way. They'll go over them, around them, or under them, which means they don't give up. They're persistent! They are always on the move—industrious, moving, saving, storing. In fact, how many couch potato ants have you seen? Of course, moving relates directly to our physical well-being and diabetes management.

Unlike Ants, We Let Obstacles Get in the Way

However, unlike ants, people let obstacles get in their way when it comes to movement. They may say things like the following: my friends and family aren't active; how would I look exercising; I don't get enough sleep as is; my free times during the day are too short; I need to walk five miles a day, but I don't have the time or energy!

Many people believe that the only way they can benefit from exercise is to intensely walk for long periods of time. I recently walked in the coolness of a mall and saw some people power walking. Is that the only way to achieve any benefits for the management of diabetes? Also, how long must one walk to get any benefit from the movement? How many steps should be taken each day? Should your goal be ten thousand steps per day?

Someone has said, "It's not what you weigh but where you weigh."

A six-month study of 464 women reported that they did an equivalent of just ten minutes of walking per day, and their waistlines shrank by nearly two inches, even when some of them didn't lose any weight.[1] Why is this so significant for people with diabetes? Research indicates the loss of visceral, or abdominal, fat can help with blood sugar management, because this fat causes an increase in insulin resistance and glucose intolerance. This fat lowers HDL cholesterol, elevates triglycerides, and contributes to hypertension.[2] Between caloric restriction and movement, the more effective way to reduce this visceral fat is through movement.[3] This reinforces the power of being wise like an ant, which among all the other attributes mentioned includes *moving!* Remember one of the excuses was, "My free times during the day are too short." It only took ten minutes a day of walking to make a difference for these women!

Someone else might say, "I'm so tired, I don't know how I could be more active each day."

A research study at the University of Georgia was done of thirty-six inactive men and women who complained of persistent fatigue. They were assigned to one of three groups. The moderate-intensity exercise group's activity consisted of walking uphill for twenty minutes, three times a week. Another group's activity was less intense and consisted of walking the same amount of time each week, but to do so leisurely. The third group had no activity. The results of this six-week study were as follows: The low intensity group reported a 65 percent drop in feelings of fatigue. The intense walking group only dropped 49 percent. Both groups had a 20 percent boost in energy. There was no change in the sedentary group.[4]

So movement, instead of draining your batteries of energy, will increase them. Obviously, this study was not done with people with diabetes and didn't examine the added factor of how high levels of blood sugar can sap you of energy. But other studies reveal that when people with diabetes move more often, their blood sugar averages come down!

Other Movement Benefits

If you were told about a once-a-day pill that could help you sleep better, restore your energy, improve your mood, reduce your risk of heart disease, help you to lose weight, and improve your blood sugar control, you would probably take it in an instant! And movement does all of that! It doesn't even stop there, because it can also increase your good cholesterol (HDL), lower your bad cholesterol (LDL), and improve blood pressure. If you have a gloomy mood, then move more. It can stimulate the brain to release endorphins, which are positive mood changers, and also release serotonin, which can stave off depression.[5]

Motivation

I want to tell you about a remarkable tool that I've found to be so helpful for moving more. More than six years ago, I lost sixteen pounds by concentrating on the amounts of all the types of foods I was eating, not just carbohydrates. A tremendous factor in my weight loss, though, was also the use of a pedometer! Even now I start my day with a pedometer in my pocket! It's easier to count steps than to count calories. You can set a goal of the number of steps you want to walk each day, and the pedometer will show you how many you have taken at any given time during the day. My goal is to take ten thousand steps per day. It helps with motivation, too. If you've only walked seven thousand steps by the evening, and your goal is ten thousand, you'll be more likely to walk to make up the difference. At least, that's been my experience.

Pedometers Prove to Increase Movement

A research study on the use of pedometers was reported in the April, 2005, issue of *American College of*

Sports Medicine Journal. The research was conducted with two groups. The participants in one group were to wear a pedometer and have a goal of ten thousand steps per day. The other group's goal was to take a brisk, thirty-minute walk per day. Both groups wore pedometers, but the pedometers worn by the brisk, thirty-minute-a-day walking group was a non-viewable one. The group using the viewable pedometers averaged over 10,000 steps per day while the thirty-minute walking group only walked an average of 8,270 steps— a difference of almost a mile per day.

What was really revealing, though, were the days the groups did not meet their goals. The pedometer 10,000-steps-per-day group still walked 7,780 steps, as opposed to 5,597 steps for the thirty-minute-a-day walk group. The pedometer group was apparently motivated to take more steps than they did before the study. The thirty-minute-a-day group, however, did not increase their steps on days they didn't take their thirty-minute walk.[6]

What is the lesson from this? You may walk forty to fifty minutes a day with a walking program, but what are you doing the rest of the day? We can become couch potatoes or yield to "sitting disease" during the rest of the day. Your pedometer will show you how many steps you are getting during those non–walking program periods. In other words, set a step goal each day, and keep stepping until you get it.

Diabetes in Control 10,000 Step Study

The value of walking with a pedometer was confirmed in the Diabetes in Control 10,000 step study. Participants who had Type 2 diabetes were to increase their steps to ten thousand per day without any change in what they ate. In this three-month study, some positive outcomes were recorded. Thirty-three percent reduced dosages of diabetes medications, 14 percent went off some of the medications, and 7 percent eliminated all medications. Average weight loss was four pounds, as a result of walking ten thousand steps per day.

Another study reported in Diabetes Care confirmed that by just adding 4,400 steps (about 2.2 miles) to what people normally walked per day a reduction in blood glucose levels, total cholesterol, triglycerides, and blood pressure was achieved. More movement, like taking ten thousand steps per day, reaps even more benefits.[7]

The following are comments from participants in the Diabetes in Control 10,000 step study on the benefits of using a pedometer:

"I reduced my stress levels." "It was very easy to just put on the pedometer and check it during the day—it really works." "I never thought I could get to ten thousand steps a day, but just by tracking my steps and increasing ten percent a week, I was able to do it!" "I was surprised to see that it became a habit after just a short time." "My whole family wanted pedometers, and they also increased their steps." "Just by removing the remote controllers, we picked up four hundred steps." "My dog is healthier than ever (I wore the pedometer, not the dog)." "I have more energy, and my blood sugars have never been better. Now my doctor is wearing a pedometer." "My blood pressure is down to normal." "My clothes all fit better."[8]

What Doctors at the Cooper Clinic Have Said about Pedometers

Dr. Tedd Mitchell wrote, "Like most doctors, I always considered myself busy and active at work. I'm up and down, and all around, seeing patients day long. I clipped on a step counter. I checked the step counter at noon, and I had taken only 500 steps over the course of four hours. It took the step counter to open my eyes to the deceptively sedentary nature of my work." Dr. Tim Church wrote, "I am always walking around the facility to peek in on studies in progress and monitor exercise testing. One day I decided to see just how much activity I accumulated in my routine workday. I put on a step counter. I logged 2,900 steps—smack in the sedentary category. What I learned was that anybody who puts on a step counter is in for a real surprise."[9]

Should Your Step Count Goal Be Ten Thousand Steps per Day?

A twenty-four-month study was done of thirty-two women between the ages of forty and sixty. First, there was a determination of the average daily steps they took, which was about 6,500. Then they were asked to add to that number two to three thousand more steps. The result was that they lowered their total cholesterol number and increased the HDL levels.

Sedentary people in the USA generally move only two to three thousand steps per day. Older adults and those living with chronic diseases typically take 3,500 to 5,500 steps per day. In one study, healthy older adults, who were sixty-nine years old and older, took about 6,600 steps per day, with almost 3,000 steps coming from structured, planned movement. This means they would have a structured walk of about one-and-a-half miles per day. Other studies have shown that moving six thousand steps a day can significantly increase health and wellness benefits, and eight to ten thousand per day promotes weight loss.[10]

Research Study at the Mayo Clinic

Why do I need a pedometer, when I can plan to walk two or three times a day? I know I can get my thirty-eight minutes of walking in that way. An extensive eight-week study in which sixteen sedentary people were fed exactly a thousand extra calories per day was done at the Mayo Clinic. It was an extra 56,000 calories that were eaten by each participant. Each person should have gained about sixteen pounds. What were the results?

One person barely gained an ounce. By contrast, one lady gained fourteen pounds! Everyone else was in between those extremes. How could some people barely gain any weight? Where were all those extra calories going? They had to be shedding all those calories just through daily life, but how? They were not allowed to start a walking program, either. No one went out and walked several miles each night.

Ethan was the guy who didn't gain any weight. How did he do it? Was he sneaking in exercise, doing a midnight marathon? No! He didn't even realize it, but he had started moving more. Instead of driving his son to the bus stop, he walked him. He started pacing up and down the sidelines during his son's soccer games. He even got up in the middle of the night and did little things, like adjust the drapes or shut the window. He didn't even remember those actions, but his wife did and told about them. Those who didn't gain weight in this Mayo Clinic overfeeding study responded by spontaneously moving more.[11]

Why does spontaneously moving help? Dr. Levine at the Mayo Clinic informs us that our capillaries are lined with special cells (endothelial), which contain an enzyme (lipoprotein lipase LPL) that breaks down fat molecules (triglycerides) in the blood. These enzymes start to switch off when we sit for a few hours. The mere act of getting up out of a chair breaks them out of hibernation mode.[12]

Suggestions on Moving More

Instead of parking your car as close to the front entrance of a store as you possibly can, why not park your car way back in the corner of the parking lot, where the people with brand new cars park theirs? It gives you the opportunity to put more steps on your pedometer. A small activity, like standing up and stretching during the commercials of a basketball or football game you're watching, can make a difference. Mowing the lawn, sweeping the sidewalk, raking leaves, walking up and down a flight of stairs, or just standing more will all help burn more calories.

After-Meal Blood Sugar Levels

A research study was done at the University of Missouri to determine the effect walking ten thousand steps a day has on post meal blood sugar levels. Blood sugar measurements were made for three days, while volunteers went about their normal routines on a ten-thousand-step-per-day regimen and then were contrasted with a routine of purposely moving less than five thousand steps per day. They ate the same amount of calories under each regimen, but with the inactivity routine, blood sugar levels would spike up after meals. In fact, they were averaging twenty-six percent higher and were trending higher on each subsequent day of inactivity. When they returned to the ten-thousand-step-per-day routine blood sugars went back down.

Get Up and Move Every Thirty Minutes

Another study was done to see the benefits for office workers of taking a two-minute exercise break every twenty minutes for blood sugar control. Think about this: if you sit at a desk, do you normally get up and move that often? Most people don't, and that's one reason it sounded to me like a novel thing to research. And sure enough, they discovered that blood sugar levels were reduced by a whopping 30 percent! I'm concluding from all of this research that it would be a good idea to be on the move more, how about you?[13]

A person weighing 150 pounds will burn 36, 71, 107 calories while walking 10, 20 or 30 minutes at a 2.5 mile pace per hour respectively. If the pace is increased to 3.0 miles per hour the calories burned will be 46, 83 or 125 while walking 10, 20 or 30 minutes respectively. To calculate how many calories you will burn based upon your specific weight go to www.caloriesburnedHQ.com. By taking shorter walks throughout the day I accumulate an average of 11,000 steps per day as well as maintain better blood glucose control.

The Way of Wisdom on Work

The way of wisdom teaches us to follow the example of the ant and be wise. One of ants' characteristics is that they are always on the move, working. Another aspect to movement is to think about work. Most of the proverbs were written about 1000 BC. How many desk jobs were there in 1000 BC? Most work was manual labor, involving shepherding sheep or planting and cultivating crops. People in that day and time were on their feet, moving more!

Suppose you were at home at three in the afternoon and received a call from your daughter, who was at a school function thirty miles away and needed a ride home. How long would the round trip take? Normally, you could be there and back by supper time. In the first century AD, there is an example from the book of Acts about three men traveling from Caesarea to Joppa, which was a distance of about thirty miles. They left their home after three o'clock in the afternoon and didn't get to Joppa until about noon the next day. Today, it would be a completely different story, because today they could get in their car and be there in just a short time. In the first century, however, they walked, and it took twenty-one hours, which probably included a time during the night to stop for sleep.

Lifestyles in the Past Required a Greater Level of Physical Activity

---

Of course, in the first century and centuries before that when these proverbs were written there would have been no modern technological conveniences. The very lifestyles of people would require a greater level of physical activity during those times. In 2004, researchers from the University of Tennessee studied the level of activity among ninety-eight participants between the ages of eighteen and seventy-five from an Old Order Amish community in southern Ontario. Their lifestyle requires that they abstain from driving automobiles, using electrical appliances or other modern conveniences. Their way of life has basically stayed the same for the last one hundred fifty years. Farming is still the predominate occupation. Participants were asked to wear a pedometer for seven days and to fill out a log sheet on which they recorded their number of steps per day and physical activities. The research was done in the month of June.

Fifty-three men and forty-five women participated and what the researchers discovered was a high level of physical activity. The Amish men reported doing an average of ten hours of vigorous activity and about forty-three hours of moderate activity per week. The women reported doing about three and a half hours of vigorous activity and thirty-nine hours of moderate activity per week. The average number of steps per day was almost stunning! The average number of steps per day was 18,425 for men versus 14,196 for women. There was no significant difference by age either.

There is a stark contrast between this community and the general population when it comes to weight. The latest statistics from the Centers for Disease Control and Prevention for the percentage of people over age twenty who are overweight and obese is 72.9 % (that is, people who have a body mass index of 25 or above). For the Old Order Amish community it was just 26 %. Obesity is prevalent in 35.9 % of the population. Obesity is defined as having a BMI greater than or equal to 30. Whereas, in this Amish community, there were only 4 % who would be considered obese.[14] (If you want to calculate your BMI just take your weight and divide it by your number of inches in height. Take the result of that calculation and divide it by your height in inches again. Then multiply that result by 703 to get the BMI.

For example, Weight = 150 lbs., Height = 5'5" (65 inches)
BMI Calculation: [150 ÷ (65)2] x 703 = 24.96)

So what we read in God's wisdom about the benefits of work is multifaceted. It is not just about financial benefits; it is about physical benefits as well. Remember the statement that these wisdom teachings *"are life to those who find them. They are health to your whole body"* (Proverbs 4:22). With all of this in mind, when we read what is stated in the following passages about work, we gain a greater depth of insight into how really beneficial work is for one's whole well-being.

"From the fruit of his lips a man is filled with good things, as surely as the work of his hands rewards him" (Proverbs 12:14). *"All hard work brings a profit, but mere talk leads only to poverty"* (Proverbs 14:23). *"I went past the field of the sluggard, past the vineyard of the man who lacks judgment; thorns had come up everywhere, the ground was covered with weeds, and the stone wall was in ruins. I applied my heart to what I observed and learned a lesson from what I saw: A little sleep, a little slumber, a little folding of the hands to rest—and poverty will come on you like a bandit and scarcity like an armed man"* (Proverbs 24:30–34).

Research Indicates the Positive Effects of Working Out

Another aspect to consider about physical activity is weight or resistance training. In the last proverb, when that person's stone wall was in ruins it would take the lifting of stones to repair it. Stones are like weights. A research study was done by the University of Calgary and the University of Ottawa on the effects of aerobic training alone, resistance training alone, and the combination of both types of exercise on the hemoglobin

A1c values in patients with type 2 diabetes. Two hundred fifty-one people with Type 2 diabetes between the ages of thirty-nine to seventy were the participants in this twenty-two week study. To qualify for the study one of the basic requirements was to basically be sedentary.

The principal measurement used to determine the effects of the three categories of exercise training was the change in the hemoglobin A1c value at six months. (Read chapter two for more information on the hemoglobin A1c test.) They were randomly selected in equal numbers to the aerobic training, resistance training, combined exercise training, and control groups. The aerobic exercise group progressed from fifteen to twenty minutes per session to forty-five minutes per session three times a week. Seven different exercises on weight machines each session were done by the resistance training group. They progressed to two to three sets of each exercise with a maximum weight that could be lifted seven to nine times. Those doing both types of exercise followed the same schedule format as the individual groups did. Those in the control group were to maintain the physical activity levels they had before being selected for the study. Initially, there was a four week run-in phase to assess adherence before the twenty-two week study began.

What were the results? They saw improvements in blood-sugar control in everyone who worked out. Participants in the aerobic group had a reduction of .51% in their hemoglobin A1c values. The weight-training group had a .38 % reduction compared with control group. When both types of exercise were done there was an additional reduction of .46 % compared to the aerobic group and a reduction of .59 % for the resistance training group.[15] That is almost a total reduction in the A1c of one percentage point, which reduces the risk of heart attack, stroke, eye and kidney complications.

Every Step Counts

Mona was fifty-four years old and had had diabetes for fifteen years. She weighed 350 pounds and knew she needed to lose weight. She also knew she needed to walk about three to five miles per day but wasn't able. She decided to start by just walking to her mailbox, rest, and then walk back. When she told her doctor of the plan, he thought it was "physiologically silly," because it would not have a noticeable effect on blood glucose, weight, or blood pressure. But she formed a habit, doing it every day; and then after a few weeks she started going to the end of the block. After one year, she made her goal of three miles per day by increasing the amount she walked each week.[16]

The Example of Raymond

One person in our diabetes support group lost 180 pounds. How did he do it? It was with another "way of wisdom" principle: "Patience and the power of the small." What about 3,500? What does it have to do with this principle? 3,500 calories equals one pound. If one eats just ten calories a day beyond what is needed, what will happen? It will result in gaining a pound of weight after one year. If a person did this for ten years, the person would have gained ten pounds. If a person consumed twenty extra calories, it would be twenty pounds. Keep doing this, and the power of the small works against you. Do the reverse, and it will work for you! If you were to cut back one hundred calories a day, you could lose ten pounds in one year.

So a slow, patient, small, methodical approach is what Raymond used to lose 180 pounds. It took him three years to lose the weight. Raymond has Type 2 diabetes and uses both Lantus insulin and Humalog. It wasn't an easy task, but he never gave up! He cut back on his calories and also started a walking program. He started small and worked his way up to walking three miles a day in the morning and then in the evening too. His efforts added up and made the difference, but it took three years!

Patience Carries a Lot of Wait!

The way of wisdom teaches the value of patience, which can help us gain better health using a slow, small, methodical approach. Keep the following in mind:

"Those who are patient have great understanding, but the quick-tempered display folly" (Proverbs 14:29). *"Dishonest money dwindles away, but he who gathers money little by little makes it grow"* (Proverbs 13:11). *"Better a patient man than a warrior, a man who controls his temper than one who takes a city"* (Proverbs 16:32). *"With patience you can convince a ruler, and a gentle word can get through to the hard-headed"* (Proverbs 25:15). Many people in our diabetes support group are using the patient approach and using pedometers. One person has lost fifty pounds, and two others have each lost more than twenty pounds. Let's keep moving, achieving our goals one step at a time!

1. James A. Levine, MD, PhD, *Move a Little, Lose a Lot: New NEAT Science Reveals How to Be Thinner, Happier, and Smarter* (New York: Crown Publishers, 2009), 29.

2. Richard Beaser, MD, ed., *Joslin Diabetes Deskbook: A Guide for Primary Care Providers* (Boston: Joslin Diabetes Center, 2010), 81–82.

3. Beaser, 86.

4. Levine, 29.

5. Richard Jackson, MD, and Amy Tenderich, *Know Your Numbers, Outlive Your Diabetes: Five Essential Health Factors You Can Master to Enjoy a Long and Healthy Life* (New York: Marlowe & Company, 2007), 104, 107.

6. Wendy Bumgardner, Pedometers Proven to Increase Exercise http://walking. about.com/od/measure/a/pedometer0405.htm (Accessed July 17, 2012).

7. Sheri R. Colberg, PhD, *The 7 Step Diabetes Fitness Plan: Living Well and Being Fit with Diabetes No Matter Your Weight* (New York: Marlowe & Company, 2006), 10, 40.

8. Diabetes In Control Step Study, http://www.diabetesincontrol.com/ index. php?option=com_content&view-article&id=2001 (Accessed July 17, 2012).

9. Tedd Mitchell, MD, Tim Church, MD, PhD, and Martin Zucker, *Move Yourself: The Cooper Clinic Medical Director's Guide to All the Healing Benefits of Exercise (Even a Little!)* (Hoboken, New Jersey: John Wiley & Sons, Inc., 2008), 115–16.

10. Catrine Tudor-Locke, PhD, and David R. Bassett, Jr., PhD, How Many Steps/ Day Are Enough? Preliminary Pedometer Indices for Public Health, http:// www.health.utah.edu/PEAK/Health_Fitness/ Tudor%20Locke%20Paper.pdf (Accessed June 20, 2012).

11. Levine, 38–43.

12. Levine, 26.

13. Diabetes Health Staff, Two Studies Confirm the Role of Exercise in Blood Glucose Control, http://www.diabeteshealth.com/read/2012/03/03/7458/ two-studies-confirm-the-role-of-exercise-in-blood-glucose-control/ (Accessed June 21, 2012).

14. David R. Bassett, Jr., PhD, Patrick L. Schneider, and Gertrude E. Huntington, Physical Activity in an Old Order Amish Community, American College of Sports Medicine, 2004 http://huffinesinstitute.org/Portals/37/Bassett_ MSSE_36_04.pdf (Accessed January 14, 2013).

15. Ronald J. Sigal, MD, MPH and Glen P. Kenny, PhD, Effects of Aerobic Training, Resistance Training, or Both on Glycemic Control in Type 2 Diabetes, Annals of Internal Medicine, Volume 147, Number 6, September 18, 2007 http:// www.jhsph.edu/sebin/g/u/9_25_07JC.pdf (Accessed January 14, 2013)

16. William H. Polonsky, PhD, *Diabetes Burnout: What to Do When You Can't Take It Anymore* (Alexandria, Virginia: American Diabetes Association, 1999), 116, 129.

Chapter 12

Eating Just the Right Amounts and Making the Best Decisions Ahead of Time

---

Having the Right Perception

I read about a lady who went into an auto parts store. She asked for a seven-ten cap. The employees all looked at each other and said, "What's a seven-ten cap?" She said, "You know, it's right on the engine. Mine got lost somehow, and I need a new one." "What kind of a car is it on?" they ask. Perhaps it was an old Datsun 710—but no, she says, "It's a Buick." "OK, lady, how big is it?" She makes a circle with her hands about 3 1/2 inches in diameter. "What does it do?" they ask. She says, "I don't know, but it's always been there."

One of the employees gives her a note pad and asks her if she can draw a picture of it. So she makes a circle about 3 1/2 inches in diameter, and in the center she writes 710. The guy behind the counter is looking at it upside down as she writes it, and it dawns on him what she is actually talking about. He says, "I think you want an oil cap." She says, "Seven-ten cap, oil cap, I don't care what you call it, I just need one!" By the way, you've probably figured it out by now, the word "OIL" upside down looks like "710."

Perception, Popcorn, and Size of Container

That example really illustrates the power of perception. How much movie theater popcorn do people eat? Does it depend on how hungry they are or how good it tastes? Could the size of the box influence how much one eats? A study was done by Dr. Wansink to determine the influence of the box size on the amount eaten. At a theater in Chicago at a 1:05 p.m. showing, people were given a free box of popcorn. Some were given a large container, and others were given a medium-sized box.

Participants were asked to answer a few concession stand questions after the movie. They were to also return their bucket or box with any uneaten popcorn. The only catch was, they were not told the popcorn had been popped five days before and was kept in sterile conditions. Participants were told, "We have found that the average person who is given a large-size container eats more than if they are given a medium-size container. Do you think you ate more because you had the large size?" Most of the participants disagreed. They thought the size of the container had no effect on the amount one would eat. The big-bucket group, however, actually ate 173 more calories than the medium-sized group. They ate 53 percent more than those with the medium-sized boxes. The conclusion was that people eat more when given a bigger container!

What would be a good application for using that information on a daily basis? If you spoon four ounces of sweet potatoes onto a twelve-inch plate, it will look like a lot less than if you had spooned it onto an eight-inch plate.[1] Why not put your food on a midsize plate instead of the larger plate, giving it the appearance of holding more food? We all need to restrict the amount of food we eat to the proper portion size. This could be an easy strategy to use to aid with that goal. The way of wisdom says, *"The wise in heart are called discerning"* (Proverbs 16:21).

Portion Control with Measurements

Someone says, "My problem is portion control. I just eat too much." "My doctor has advised me to give up those intimate little dinners for four, unless there are three other people with me"—Orson Welles. The way of wisdom principle is portion control. Wisdom's way says, *"If you find honey, eat just enough"* (Proverbs 25:16). *"If you sit down to eat with a ruler, notice the food that is in front of you. Control yourself if you have a big appetite"* (Proverbs 23:1-2). Self-control and thinking about the consequences are also components of this principle. *"Like a city whose walls are broken through is a person who lacks self-control"* (Proverbs 25:28). *"Wise people see danger and go to a safe place. But childish people keep going and suffer for it"* (Proverbs 22:3). Remember, if you want to maintain your current weight, multiply your weight by eleven to get your total calorie ceiling for the day. For example, if you weigh two hundred pounds, multiply that number by eleven to get your calorie ceiling of 2200 calories per day.[2]

According to the Joslin Diabetes Center, the amount of carbohydrate consumption matters for diabetes management. When carbohydrate consumption is reduced from 55 percent to 40 percent of the daily amount of food, visceral fat is reduced, and insulin sensitivity improves.[3]

Measure Your Food

One of the best tools I've used to help with portion control is to use a gram scale. I've been using the EatSmart™ Digital Nutrition Scale, which calculates carbs, fiber, and fats. You can enter a code or identifying number of a certain food, like apples, which is 002, and get the total calorie count. After first removing the core and placing the apple on the scale, one can learn the total calories, grams of carbohydrate, and grams of fiber. There is a database with nutritional values for a thousand foods.

By using a tool like this, the guesswork can be removed and replaced with accuracy, which is especially important when counting carbs for the amount of insulin to inject. I like how it gives the exact amount of fiber too. On food labels, fiber is counted in the total number of carbohydrate grams. Fiber, however, is actually a complex carbohydrate that the body can't break down. It has several benefits such as helping to prevent blood glucose spikes after a meal, control food cravings, give a longer lasting full feeling and helps with weight control since more volume of food is eaten with less calories. So, how much fiber do we need in order to reap the benefits? According to the American Dietetic Association twenty to thirty-five grams are recommended per day, and of that, 5 – 10 grams should be soluble fiber. Americans only get about 15 or less grams of total fiber per day. Drink plenty of water per day (64 ounces) because fiber works best when it absorbs water.[4]

There are two types of fiber: insoluble and soluble. Insoluble fiber absorbs water, but does not dissolve in it. Insoluble fiber is found in such foods as bran flakes, bran muffins and whole wheat bread. Soluble fiber dissolves in water and becomes a gummy gel, which slows down the absorption of glucose and helps blunt elevated blood glucose after a meal. Soluble fiber is found in such foods as apples, citric fruits, oat bran, oatmeal, dried beans and peas.[5] For example, Bob's Red Mill™ Oat Bran cereal has 7 grams of fiber per serving of which 2 grams is soluble fiber. Bob's Red Mill™ Rolled Oats cereal has 5 grams of fiber per serving which includes 1.6 grams soluble fiber.

From information supplied by Harvard University Health Services, I've selected a list of foods which are especially rich in soluble fiber and should be included in our meal plans.[6] Each food is listed with serving size, then total fiber grams per serving and the number of grams of soluble fiber included in each serving. Cooked Vegetables: Asparagus ½ cup 2.8, 1.7 Broccoli ½ cup 2.4, 1.2 Brussels sprouts ½ cup 3.8, 2.0 Carrots, sliced ½ cup 2.0, 1.1 Okra, frozen ½ cup 4.1, 1.0 Peas, green, frozen ½ cup 4.3, 1.3 Sweet Potato, flesh only ½ cup 4.0, 1.8 Turnip ½ cup 4.8, 1.7 Raw Vegetables: Carrots, fresh 1, 7 ½ in. long 2.3, 1.1 Celery, fresh 1 cup chopped 1.7, 0.7 Onion, fresh ½ cup chopped 1.7, 0.9 Pepper, green, fresh 1 cup chopped 1.7, 0.7 Fruits: Apple, red, fresh w/skin 1 small 2.8, 1.0 Apricots, dried 7 halves 2.0, 1.1 Apricots, 4 fresh w/skin 3.5, 1.8 Figs, dried 1 ½ 3.0, 1.4 Grapefruit, fresh ½ medium 1.6, 1.1 Kiwifruit, fresh, flesh only 1 large 1.7, 0.7 Orange, fresh, flesh only 1 small 2.9, 1.8 Peach, fresh, w/skin 1 medium 2.0, 1.0 Pear, fresh, w/skin ½ large 2.9, 1.1 Plum, red, fresh 2 medium 2.4, 1.1 Prunes, dried 3 medium 1.7, 1.0 Raspberries, fresh 1 cup 3.3, 0.9 Strawberries, fresh 1 ¼ cup 2.8, 1.1 Legumes (cooked): Black beans ½ cup 6.1, 2.4 Black-eyed peas ½ cup 4.7, 0.5 Chick peas, dried ½ cup 4.3, 1.3 Kidney beans, light red ½ cup 7.9, 2.0 Lentils ½ cup 5.2, 0.6 Lima beans ½ cup 4.3, 1.1 Navy beans ½ cup 6.5, 2.2 Pinto beans ½ cup 6.1, 1.4 Breads and Crackers: Pumpernickel 1 slice 2.7, 1.2 Rye 1 slice 1.8, 0.8

When counting carbs should the fiber be counted as well? To get the net amount of carbs to count recommendations vary from subtracting all of the fiber to subtracting half of the fiber when it is more than five grams per serving.[7] From my own experience with my CGM (continuous glucose monitoring system, which gives glucose results every five minutes transmitted to my insulin pump from interstitial tissue), subtracting all the fiber when it is about five or less seems to make little difference in blood glucose levels.

Whatever the fiber content is, however, it should be subtracted from the total carbohydrate amount for each serving! This is especially important if you are using insulin. It can make a pronounced impact on the glucose levels when only half the fiber is subtracted because of the carb to insulin ratio, which I've described in chapter nine. I tried this for breakfast with All-Bran™ cereal on two consecutive mornings. A serving size of All-Bran™ is twenty-three grams with ten of that being fiber. So I subtracted all of the fiber one morning and half the fiber the next morning. I used my carb to insulin ratio (1 unit covers 9 grams of carbs for my early morning ratio). Obviously on the morning I only subtracted half the fiber grams I gave more insulin. So on the first morning when I subtracted all the fiber my BG was 73, my insulin dose was 2.3 units (13 grams of carbs in the cereal plus 10 grams in the milk) and two hours later my BG was 126, which was very good! The next morning I followed the same guidelines except I started higher with BG at 98, counted 18 grams of carb in the cereal (subtracting only half the fiber plus 10 grams of carb in the milk). My insulin dose was 3.1 since the BG started higher and I counted more carbs in the cereal. Two hours later my BG was 95 and quickly falling. Based upon my experience I recommend subtracting all the fiber rather than just half to get the net carbohydrates in a serving. Test it yourself on various carbohydrates with fiber. See what kind of blood glucose results you will have as well. Checking it yourself will be the wise thing to do! "The simple believe anything, but the prudent give thought to their steps" (Proverbs 14:15).

Also if you are trying to lose weight eating food rich in fiber will be to your advantage since you can eat more volume of food, but without having to count the fiber grams (4 calories per gram). I used this method several years ago and lost sixteen pounds. For example, a serving of All-Bran™ cereal has .5 grams of polyunsaturated fat (5 calories), 4 grams of protein (16 calories) and 23 grams of carbohydrate (92 calories) which results in a 113 total calories. But when the 10 grams of fiber listed under the carbohydrates is subtracted the total is 73 calories (10 grams of fiber x 4 calories per gram is 40 calories subtracted). Apparently, Kellogg's All-Bran™ has already done this since the total calories listed per serving are 80 calories. Many food labels, however do not automatically subtract the fiber so be sure and examine the label carefully.

When looking at a food label, also note under the total carbohydrates that some are listed as sugar alcohol. Sugar alcohols are digested very slowly and only partially. Count only half what is listed when counting carbs. Sugar alcohols are found in many low-fat, low-carb ice creams.[8]

Glycemic Index (GI) and Glycemic Load (GL)

All carbohydrates are not the same when it comes to affecting your blood sugar control. White rice and potatoes tend to spike up blood sugars, whereas black beans and even sweet potatoes have a different effect. One way to think of this is that heavy rain can cause flooding, while gentle rain is good for the garden. The lower the glycemic index number of a food, the more like the gentle rain metaphor it is when it comes to keeping blood glucose levels in check.

What kinds of carbohydrates raise blood glucose levels least? Numbers have been assigned based on research on how fast a particular carbohydrate will make blood glucose rise in a two-hour period, compared to an equal quantity of pure glucose. All carbohydrates are compared to glucose, which is given the base line number of 100. The smaller the number is, the better the results will be for maintaining good blood glucose levels. The glycemic load (GL) number is for the "typical" serving. The result of each food can be seen by going to www.glycemicindex.com. The results are put into the following three categories, which are based on the glycemic index number:

High: 70 and up (>20 GL). Examples include broken rice, white, cooked (86 Glycemic Index, 37 Glycemic Load, 1 cup serving, 43 Carbohydrate grams), donut, cake type (76 GI, 17 GL, 1.75 oz, 23 Carb grams), English muffin (77 GI, 11 GL, 1 oz, 14 Carb grams), French fries, frozen, reheated in microwave (75 GI, 22 GL, 30 pcs, 29 Carb grams), instant potato, mashed (97 GI, 17 GL, ¾ cup, 20 Carb grams), instant rice, white, cooked 6 min (87 GI, 36 GL, ¾ cup, 42 Carb grams), Life Savers™ (70 GI, 21 GL, 18 pcs, 30 Carb grams), popcorn, plain, cooked in microwave oven (72 GI, 8 GL, 1 ½ cups, 11 Carb grams), potato, baked (85 GI, 26 GL, 5 oz, 30 Carb grams), potato, microwaved (82 GI, 27 GL, 5 oz, 33 Carb grams), premium soda crackers (74 GI, 12 GL, 5 crackers, 17 Carb grams), pretzels (83 GI, 16 GL, 1 oz, 20 Carb grams), puffed rice cakes, white (82 GI, 17 GL, 3 cakes, 21 Carb grams), pumpkin (75 GI, 3 GL, 3 oz, 4 Carb grams), red-skinned potato, peeled and microwaved on high for 6 to 7.5 min (79 GI, 14 GL, 5 oz, 18 Carb grams), red-skinned potato, peeled, boiled 35 min (88 GI, 16 GL, 5 oz, 18 Carb grams), red-skinned potato, peeled, mashed (91 GI, 18 GL, 5 oz, 20 Carb grams), Rice Krispies™ (82 GI, 22 GL, 1 ¼ cup, 26 Carb grams), Shredded Wheat™ (75 GI, 15 GL, 2/3 cup, 20 Carb grams), Total™ (76 GI, 17 GL, ¾ cup, 22 Carb grams), watermelon (72 GI, 4 GL, 4 oz, 6 Carb grams), Wheaties™ (82 GI, 17 GL, 1 cup, 21 Carb grams), white bread (70 GI, 10 GL, 1 oz, 14 Carb grams), white rice, instant, cooked 6 min (87 GI, 36 GL, 1 cup, 42 Carb grams), whole-wheat bread (77 GI, 9 GL, 1 oz, 12 Carb grams).

Medium: 56 to 69 (11 to 19). Examples include apricots, fresh, 3 medium (57 GI, 5 GL, 4 oz serving, 9 Carb grams), cantaloupe, fresh (65 GI, 4 GL, 4 oz, 6 Carb grams), grapes, black, fresh (59 GI, 11 GL, ¾ cup,

18 Carb grams), kiwi fruit, (58 GI, 7 GL, 4 oz, 12 Carb grams), long-grain rice, cooked 10 min (61 GI, 22 GL, 1 cup, 36 Carb grams), macaroni and cheese, made from mix (64 GI, 32 GL, 1 cup, 51 Carb grams), oatmeal, cooked 1 min (66 GI, 17 GL, 1 cup, 26 Carb grams), pancakes, prepared from mix (67 GI, 39 GL, 2 4" pancakes, 58 Carb grams), pita bread, white (57 GI, 10 GL, 1 oz, 17 Carb grams), pizza, cheese (60 GI, 16 GL, 1 slice, 27 Carb grams), pineapple, fresh (66 GI, 6 GL, 4 oz, 10 Carb grams), Raisin Bran™ (61 GI, 12 GL, ½ cup, 19 Carb grams), raisins (64 GI, 28 GL, ½ cup, 44 Carb grams), rye bread (58 GI, 8 GL, 1 oz, 14 Carb grams), spaghetti, durum wheat, cooked 20 min (64 GI, 27 GL, 1 ½ cups, 43 Carb grams), Special K™ (69 GI, 14 GL, 1 cup, 21 Carb grams), taco shells, baked (68 GI, 8 GL, 2 shells, 12 Carb grams), tortilla chips, plain, salted (63 GI, 17 GL, 1.75 oz, 26 Carb grams).

Low: 55 and under (<10 GL). Examples include All-Bran™ cereal (30 GI, 4 GL, ½ cup serving, 15 Carb grams), apple, fresh, medium (38 GI, 6 GL, 4 oz, 15 Carb grams), banana, fresh, medium (52 GI, 12 GL, 4 oz, 24 Carb grams), barley, pearled, cooked (25 GI, 11 GL, 1 cup, 42 Carb grams), black beans, cooked (30 GI, 7 GL, 4/5 cup, 23 Carb grams), black-eyed peas, canned (42 GI, 7 GL, 2/3 cup, 17 Carb grams), brown rice, cooked (50 GI, 16 GL, 1 cup, 33 Carb grams), butter beans, canned (31 GI, 6 GL, 2/3 cup 20 Carb grams), carrots, peeled, cooked (49 GI, 2 GL, ½ cup, 5 Carb grams), carrots, raw (47 GI, 3 GL, 1 medium, 6 Carb grams), cherries, fresh (22 GI, 3 GL, 18 cherries, 12 Carb grams), chickpeas or garbanzo beans, canned (42 GI, 9 GL, 2/3 cup, 22 Carb grams), chickpeas, dried, cooked (28 GI, 8 GL, 2/3 cup, 30 Carb grams), dates, dried, (50 GI, 20 GL, 7 dates, 40 Carb grams), French green beans, cooked (0 GI, 0 GL, ½ cup, 0 Carb grams), grapefruit, fresh, medium (25 GI, 3 GL, 1 half, 11 Carb grams), grapes, green, fresh (46 GI, 8 GL, ¾ cup, 18 Carb grams), green peas (48 GI, 3 GL, 1/3 cup, 7 Carb grams), honey (55 GI, 10 GL, 1 Tbsp, 18 Carb grams), kidney beans, canned (52 GI, 9 GL, 2/3 cup, 17 Carb grams), kidney beans, cooked (23 GI, 6 GL, 2/3 cup, 25 Carb grams), 28, 7), lentils, brown, cooked (29 GI, 5 GL, ¾ cup, 18 Carb grams), lentils, red, cooked, (26 GI, 5 GL, ¾ cup, 18 Carb grams), lima beans, baby, frozen (32 GI, 10 GL, ¾ cup 30 Carb grams), macaroni, cooked (GI 47, GL 23, 1 ¼ cup, 48 Carb grams), mango (51 GI, 8 GL, 4 oz, 15 Carb grams), navy beans, canned (38 GI, 12 GL, 5 oz, 31 Carb grams), peach, fresh, large (42 GI, 5 GL, 4 oz, 11 Carb grams), peanuts (14 GI, 1 GL, 1.75 oz, 6 Carb grams), pear halves, canned in natural juice (43 GI, 5 GL, ½ cup, 13 Carb grams), pear, fresh (38 GI, 4 GL, 4 oz, 11 Carb grams), peas, green, frozen, cooked (48 GI, 3 GL, ½ cup, 7 Carb grams), pinto beans, canned (45 GI, 10 GL, 2/3 cup, 22 Carb grams), pinto beans, dried, cooked (39 GI, 10 GL, ¾ cup, 26 Carb grams), pizza, super supreme, pan 11.4% fat (36 GI, 9 GL, 1 slice, 24 Carb grams), pizza, super supreme, thin and crispy 13.2% fat (30 GI, 7 GL, 1 slice, 22 Carb grams – **read chapter nine on how fatty foods can increase blood glucose levels**), plums, fresh (39 GI, 5 GL, 2 medium, 12 Carb grams), prunes, pitted (29 GI, 10 GL, 6 prunes, 33 Carb grams), pudding, instant, vanilla, made with whole milk (40 GI, 10 GL, ½ cup, 24 Carb grams), ravioli, meat-filled, cooked (39 GI, 15 GL, 6.5 oz, 38 Carb grams), rolled oats (42 GI, 9 GL, 1 cup, 21 Carb grams), seeded rye bread (55 GI, 7 GL, 1 oz, 13 Carb grams), sourdough rye (48 GI, 6 GL, 1 oz, 12 Carb grams), sourdough wheat (54 GI, 8 GL, 1 oz, 14 Carb grams), spaghetti, white, cooked 5 min (38 GI, 18 GL, 1 ½ cups, 48 Carb grams), spaghetti, whole wheat, cooked 5 min (32 GI, 14 GL, 1 ½ cups,

44 Carb grams), split peas, yellow, cooked 20 min (32 GI, 6 GL, ¾ cup, 19 Carb grams), strawberries, fresh (40 GI, 1 GL, 4 oz, 3 Carb grams), sweet corn, whole kernel, canned, diet-pack, drained (46 GI, 13 GL, 1 cup, 28 Carb grams), sweet potato, cooked (44 GI, 11 GL, 5 oz, 25 Carb grams), tomato, chopped (28 GI, 2 GL, 1 cup, 8 Carb grams).[9]

After considering this information, a meal plan strategy can be based on the types of carbohydrates to primarily eat and the amounts. When the glycemic index number is determined, the glycemic load (typical serving size) can be calculated with the following formula: (GI value) x (available, that is, minus fiber, carbohydrate grams per serving) / (100) = glycemic load. For example, one serving of old-fashioned rolled oats has a GI of 42 x 21 (serving size of carbohydrate grams) = 882 / 100 = 8.82, which is a low-level glycemic load. However, if two servings were eaten, the result would be in the medium glycemic load range (GI of 42 x 42 = 1764 / 100 = 17.64). Obviously, the more that is eaten, the greater the impact on blood glucose levels.

In a landmark study on blood glucose control, at least it was a landmark study for me, I used my continuous glucose monitoring system with my Medtronic 530g pump with somewhat surprising results. The carbs to eat for breakfast were based on the glycemic index. For several mornings in a row I ate at the same time and ate the same amount of grams of carbohydrate, using grapefruit (GI 25, 27 grams carb with 4 grams fiber, GL 5.75), Bob's Red Mill™ extra thick rolled oats (GI 42, 27 grams carb with 4 grams fiber, GL 9.66), Bob's Red Mill™ high fiber oat bran (GI 55, 31 grams carb with 8 grams fiber, GL 12.65), sourdough wheat bread (GI 54 with no fiber, but 4 grams of butter, GL 12.42), Rice Krispies™ (GI 82, 23 grams, GL 18.86). I had one egg with each meal (two with the bread) and about a half cup of 1% milk (GI 34, 4 grams, GL 1.36) or 4 grams of carb with each meal. I subtracted all the fiber from the total carbohydrate amount and used the same amount of insulin based upon my insulin to carb ratio.

With these low glycemic load servings blood glucose was elevated from 41 points with the sourdough bread to 56 points with Rice Krispies.™ All blood glucose levels began to noticeably drop ninety minutes after eating with the exception of Rice Krispies,™ which remained at its peak level much longer. I know this is not a large scale scientific study, but it is something you can do with a glucose meter using the glycemic index as a guide. What is the lesson? Smaller serving size is the answer for blood glucose control. In comparison just consider highway traffic. When a small number of automobiles are on a given stretch of highway the traffic acts in a manageable way. Cars can maintain speed, enter and merge into open spaces, and exit with a minimum of danger. Double the number of cars and the traffic becomes more congested and unpredictable. When the amount of carbs is doubled blood glucose levels become less manageable because the glycemic load increases (for example, the Rice Krispies™ with the 18.86 GL). To make blood glucose levels more predictable eat smaller amounts of carbohydrates at each meal. It is recommended that you keep the glycemic load of your meal at or under 25.[10] "The wisdom of the prudent is to give thought to their ways, but the folly of fools is deception" (Proverbs 14:8).

The glycemic index should be used by everyone for counting carbohydrates. As previously mentioned, 40 percent of total calorie consumption should be carbohydrates each day. That means that if a person were on a 2,000 calorie meal plan, 200 grams would be carbohydrates. Why not use the glycemic index (GI) information to help determine what kinds of carbs to eat? Substitute sweet corn, which has a GI of 46 and a glycemic load of 13, for white rice, which has a GI of 87 and a GL of 36 (or, better yet, choose pearled barley, with a GI of 25 and a GL of 11). Using this combination of GI with carb counting will help with blood glucose control, which can be checked two hours after starting to eat. When counting the total carbs for calculating the amount of insulin to take, remember to subtract the grams of fiber from the total number of carbs. In the previous listing of foods, the fiber has already been subtracted to get the net Carb grams for each food.

For more examples of fiber content in foods go to www.calorieking.com and of course look at the package label for those foods that are packaged. Also use a digital scale like the EatSmart™ Digital Nutrition Scale which I mentioned at the beginning of this chapter, which gives the amount of total calories as well as the number of grams of carbohydrate and fiber for the particular food being weighed.

According to Nora Saul, manager of nutritional education at the Joslin Diabetes Center, a simple way of lowering the GI of starches is to cook them al dente, that is, for a shorter time (don't overcook, not overly soft, chewy). This prevents the swelling or gelatinization of the starch molecules. The less gelatinized (swollen) the starch is, the slower the rate of digestion, and the lower the GI value of the food and the impact it has on blood glucose (sugar) levels.

Adding an acid or fat will also help lower the GI. Acids in foods slow down stomach emptying, thereby slowing the rate at which the starch can be digested. The acids in the following examples are what can be used: vinegar, lemon juice, lime juice, some salad dressings, pickled vegetables, and sourdough bread. Healthy fats such as olive oil and nuts will also slow stomach emptying, retarding enzyme digestion. Carbohydrates that are high in fiber—especially soluble fiber, such as beans, peas, apples, oats, or Brussels sprouts—will be the best carbs to eat and contribute to better blood glucose control.[11]

Research Study of Thirty-Nine Overweight Adults Reported by the ADA

Researchers placed thirty-nine overweight or obese adults on one of two energy-restricted diets. One was a low–glycemic load diet, and the other was a low-fat diet. Resting energy expenditure (REE), the rate at which energy is expended while at rest, was used to measure outcomes.

The low-GL meal plan group showed several advantages over the low-fat meal plan group. There were improvements in insulin resistance, serum triglycerides, C-reactive protein, and blood pressure. The REE decreased less among the low-GL group than among those in the low-fat group. This was good news, because typically, the REE decreases during energy-restricted diets and thus slows down potential weight loss. According to Allison B. Goldfine, MD, co-investigator of the study and researcher at the Joslin Diabetes Center in Boston, the low-GL group also experienced less hunger.[12]

Simple Way versus Wisdom's Way

Someone might say, "I've been reading that I should have a low-carbohydrate, high-protein meal plan to keep my blood sugars in control." What he's read is right, if the carbohydrates are high on the GI scales. We've learned to count carbs and eat the right kinds of carbs to keep blood sugar under control!

The way of wisdom teaches the following: *"Be sure you know the condition of your flocks, give careful attention to your herds"* (Proverbs 27:23). The principle is to know the condition of what you own, including your body. In other words, it is a good idea to keep track of what you eat. It is also appropriate to give thought to what you do, which would include what you eat. *"The wisdom of the prudent is to give thought to their ways"* (Proverbs 14:8). *"A simple man believes anything, but a prudent man gives thought to his steps"* (Proverbs 14:15). It also teaches about portion control. *"The best food and olive oil are stored up in the houses of wise people. But a foolish man eats up everything he has"* (Proverbs 21:20).

Healthy Principle of Diligence

Diligence is needed for optimal control. Carefully read the following words concerning the way of wisdom: *"Listen, my son, accept what I say, and the years of your life will be many. I guide you in the way of wisdom and lead you along straight paths....My son, pay attention to what I say; listen closely to my words. Do not let them out of your sight, keep them within your heart; for they are life to those who find them and health to a man's whole body"* (Proverbs 4:10–11, 4:20–22). The good news is that these instructions are given to us because we are capable of keeping them!

Included in these teachings is the principle of diligence. The concept of diligence is described in the following proverbs: *"The sluggard craves and gets nothing, but the desires of the diligent are fully satisfied"* (Proverbs 13:4). *"A sluggard does not plow in season; so at harvest time he looks but finds nothing"* (Proverbs 20:4). Actually, diligence, according to the way of wisdom, is the "decide ahead of time" principle.

Most people think they know what diligence means, but do they know what it means based on God's timeless wisdom principles? It is a rare quality, because it goes against natural inclinations. A common characteristic of many people is to want as much as they can get, as fast as they can get it, with as little effort and planning as possible. In other words, this common inclination is called *instant gratification*. Someone can offer a pill for losing weight, and you have to change nothing except buy and take the pill. You end up losing something called money in this deal, but not weight.

Thinking Ahead of Time about What You Will Do

A trait that goes hand in hand with this is following the path of least resistance. It's easy to sit down in front of the TV in the evening with a bag of potato chips. How many will you eat? Will you eat as many as there are in the bag? This is the path of least resistance. Those who follow this path wouldn't even think of asking the following questions, much less of answering them: Do you always have a snack while watching TV? Is a second or third helping for a meal automatic? Do you eat before bed? Do you skip breakfast and overeat later in the day? Do most of your leisure-time activities entail sitting and eating? How many nights a week do you eat takeout, delivery, or drive-through? Do you routinely take the elevator to go less than three floors?

How many hours a day do you spend sitting down? To answer those questions, reflection is required; and then, if corrections need to be made, plans or thinking ahead of what you will do is needed!

Those who follow the wisdom trait of diligence choose to follow a path of planning, which reaps great rewards. The thesaurus has the following synonyms for diligence: hard-working, industrious, persistent, unrelenting, and tireless. Those are good terms, but they don't fully describe what the way of wisdom teaches about diligence.

For example, I may end up with a high blood sugar reading, because at a church potluck meal I eat too much tasty casserole, potatoes, and bread—and may even eat some very enticing, delicious-looking pie. Then I realize that I need to work hard and be unrelenting at bringing my blood sugar down to normal levels by taking a correction dose of fast-acting insulin like Humalog and walking. If you aren't on fast-acting insulin, walk and avoid carbohydrates during the next few hours. That would be prudent, but it would not be wisdom's definition of diligence. Diligence has more to do with working *smart* than working hard. It has to do with planning ahead for what you will do in any circumstance. It is true that diligence would involve planning what you will do to treat high blood sugar after a meal, but more importantly, it would involve planning ahead to eat the proper amounts, so that you avoid the high blood sugar in the first place.

Diligence is associated with planning in the following passages: *"A lazy man does not roast his prey, but the precious possession of a man is diligence"* (Proverbs 12:27). *"The plans of the diligent lead to profit as sure as haste leads to poverty"* (Proverbs 21:5). Another way to word this is, "The plans of the planner lead to profit."

Diligence is used in several Bible passages with the idea of cut, quick and decisive, or determined before the situation arises. Something that is cut cannot be uncut. The decision is made ahead of time, and thus what to do can be determined quickly, because the decision has already been made before the situation arises. No distraction would carry the person off course. (Read 2 Samuel 5:23–24 and 1 Kings 20:40 for more examples of the use of the word *diligence*. In 2 Samuel 5:24 the word is translated "move quickly" or "act promptly" or "act decisively" because the decision has already been made.)

"Eat honey, my son, for it is good; honey from the comb is sweet to your taste. Know also that wisdom is sweet to your soul; if you find it, there is a future hope for you, and your hope will not be cut off" (Proverbs 24:13–14).

In this proverb, the sweetness of wisdom is being described by using a comparison with honey. Honey is a low glycemic index carbohydrate (55 GI). As we know, honey is a very tasty, delicious carbohydrate. When we think of wisdom, it too should be thought of as tasty and satisfying, because it gives us hope for our lives. The following is an example of how diligence is such a very healthy (and, in a sense, tasty) wisdom principle that was effectively used in the life of a young man.

It was around Thanksgiving, 1914, when James Havens was diagnosed with what we today call Type 1 diabetes. He was almost fifteen years old. From that day on, the wisdom principle of diligence was intensely used for him. It was used during the next seven-and-a-half years to just keep him alive. He continued to use it for the next thirty-eight years until he died, not of diabetes, but colon cancer! The idea of diligence, of deciding ahead of time what to do, was followed by his mother, for she meticulously weighed every morsel of food he ate.

As mentioned in chapter 3, he was a very fortunate person, as he became the first American to receive insulin. Before insulin, however, the only therapy was Dr. Frederick Allen's "under-nutrition therapy." Dr. Allen advocated serious dieting to patients, whose complaints were their extreme hunger and rapid weight loss. The doctor seemed to be telling them that they needed to be hungry more often to keep blood sugar levels from skyrocketing higher, eventually leading to coma. This is what Jim endured for almost eight years, until he received insulin, which was discovered in the summer of 1921.

When he was diagnosed, he was almost fifteen years old and weighed ninety-seven pounds. From Thanksgiving, 1914, to May 21, 1922, he went from ninety-seven pounds to less than seventy-four pounds. During that time, he endured a meal plan of about 820 calories per day, with painstaking efforts to eliminate most carbohydrates from his meal plan.[13] Diligence, deciding ahead of time was required. By doing this, he had lived longer than anyone else on this "under-nutrition therapy."

His dad was always looking and inquiring if any new treatments were available to improve his son's life and keep him alive. He was the head of the legal department at the Eastman Kodak Company in Rochester, New York. He had combed the United States for eight years, looking for a promising treatment, but none was found. In fact, in March of 1921, his father wrote, "His condition is not such as to hold out any hope."[14]

One day George Snowball, a manager of the Kodak store in Toronto, Canada, came into his office. Mr. Havens asked if he knew anyone in Canada who was working on a cure for diabetes. He didn't, but he would inquire when he got back home. This man began to ask around and eventually discovered that Dr. Banting and his assistant, Charles Best, had made an important discovery at the University of Toronto. Of course, it was what became known as *insulin*. When Jim's dad received this exciting news, he persuaded his son's doctor, John Williams, to go to Toronto. While there, Williams was able to get some insulin from Dr. Banting.

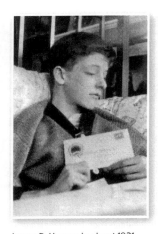

James D. Havens in about 1921 before he became the first American to receive insulin. Photo courtesy of The Thomas Fisher Rare Book Library, University of Toronto.

By May 1922, the only thing Jim could do was moan with excruciating pain. He was barely able to lift his head from his pillow. He was ready for his life to end. In fact, on his hospital chart, it was recorded that he was "anxious to die and end his misery."[15] He could bear it no longer. Over the next few days, his whole outlook was in for a dramatic change. A small amount of unrefined insulin was brought back to Rochester by Dr. Williams. On the evening of May 21, injections of insulin were started, but they seemed to have no effect.

The next week, George Snowball stopped in to see Jim's dad at Eastman Kodak. When he asked about how Jim was doing, he was surprised to hear his dad say, "I guess we're through." "But those fellows have saved lives," Snowball said.[16] Suddenly Mr. Havens shot up out of his seat and said, "George, get one of those young men over here." Mr. Snowball went to Dr. Banting and pleaded with him to go to New York, but he refused. He refused until Snowball said, "The Havens' physician tried your preparation, and it didn't work. They think it's just another failure."

Dr. Banting went to Rochester, and this time Jim received larger doses of insulin. They were given at two-hour intervals, and then the urine was checked for sugar content. Eventually, after several doses, the result was a euphoric absence of sugar in the urine. The insulin was working!

For more than seven years, Jim had been using the wisdom principle of diligence for his meal plan, and now he would continue to do so with both his eating and his daily insulin doses. We, too, have access to this powerful principle of diligence from the way of wisdom. As a result, we'll be rewarded for using it, which will then reinforce its repeated use in our lives.

How to Use the Wisdom Principle of Diligence

How can we put this powerful principle into action? First, determine how many calories you will eat each day. To maintain your current weight, multiply your weight by eleven, and the result is the number of calories you should eat each day to not gain weight. If you desire to lose weight, subtract 500 calories from that total.[17]

Glenn was telling his friend Ricky that there is nothing like getting up at sunrise, having a delicious breakfast, taking an invigorating walk around the park and then taking a refreshing shower! Ricky said, "I didn't know you got up so early every day and took invigorating walks around the park. How long have you been doing that?" Glenn sheepishly replied, "I start tomorrow." Determine how many steps you will take each day and start taking them today. A good goal to reach is ten thousand steps per day. That should be your goal, not your beginning. Be sure and take some of those steps every thirty minutes to help with blood sugar control, which we discussed in chapter 11.

Determine how many carbohydrates you should eat for each meal. How many grams of carbohydrate should there be for a 2,000 calorie meal plan? Research indicates that if carbohydrate intake is reduced to 40 percent of total calories (which would be 200 grams a day from our example), that a reduction in visceral fat will occur, and insulin sensitivity will improve. If protein is increased to about 20–30 percent of daily calorie consumption, it will result in further weight loss, along with a decrease in triglycerides and an increase in HDL. Also keep the saturated fats to less than 10 percent of total calories.[18]

Before eating out, go to the restaurant's website, look at the menu, and determine what you will eat and how much before even going. This is a practical application of diligence and will help keep you from being distracted or enticed with other food on the menu while waiting to be served. Remember, *"Let your eyes look straight ahead, fix your gaze directly before you. Make level paths for your feet and take only ways that are firm"* (Proverbs 4:25–26). According to the way of wisdom, when this is done, you will be rewarded!

When used properly, the principles of the way of wisdom will continually bring rewards for your health and wellness! Why? Because this wisdom comes from God, and He says you will be rewarded when facing challenges in all areas of your life, including your health and wellness. They will empower you to manage or even outsmart diabetes!

"Instruct the wise and they will be wiser still; teach the righteous and they will add to their learning. The fear of the LORD is the beginning of wisdom, and knowledge of the Holy One is understanding. For through wisdom your days will be many, and years will be added to your life. If you are wise, your wisdom will reward you" (Proverbs 9:9–12).

1. Brian Wansink, PhD, *Mindless Eating: Why We Eat More than We Think* (New York: Bantam Dell, 2007), 66.

2. Robert Buynak, MD, *Dr. Buynak's 1-2-3 Diabetes Diet: A Step-by-Step Approach to Weight Loss without Gimmicks or Risks* (Alexandria, Virginia: American Diabetes Association, 2006), 85.

3. Richard Beaser, MD, ed., Joslin Diabetes Deskbook: A Guide for Primary Care Providers (Boston: Joslin Diabetes Center, 2010), 87.

4. The Cleveland Clinic (2010). Improving Your Health with Fiber. http://my.clevelandclinic.org/healthy_living/nutrition/hic_improving_your_health_with_fiber.aspx (Accessed May 8, 2014).

5. Beaser, 102.

6. Harvard University Health Services (2004) Fiber Content of Foods in Common Portions. http://huhs.harvard.edu/assets/File/OurServices/Service_Nutrition_Fiber.pdf (Accessed May 14, 2014).

7. Stephanie Dunbar, MPH, RD, Esther F. Myers, PhD, RD, FADA, reviewers, Choose Your Foods: Exchange Lists for Diabetes (Alexandria, VA: American Diabetes Association, Chicago: Academy of Nutrition and Dietetics, 2008), 54.

8. Gary Scheiner, *The Ultimate Guide to Accurate Carb Counting* (New York: Marlowe & Company, 2006), 30–33.

9. Jennie Brand-Miller, PhD, Kaye Foster-Powell, and Rick Mendosa, *What Makes My Blood Glucose Go Up . . . and Down?: And 101 Other Frequently Asked Questions About Your Blood Glucose Levels* (New York: Marlowe & Company, 2003), 173-182.

10. Meri Raffetto, RD, LDN, The Glycemic Index Diet for Dummies (Hoboken, NJ: Wiley Publishing, Inc., 2010), 54, 111.

11. Nora Saul, MS, RD, LDN, CDE, Using the Glycemic Index & Glycemic Load http://blog.joslin.org/2011/05/using-the-glycemic-index-glycemic-load/ (Accessed July 17, 2012).

12. Elizabeth Heubeck, Research Shows Benefit of Low–Glycemic-Load Diet Over Low-Fat Diet http://docnews.diabetesjournals.org/content/2/6/10.full (Accessed July 17, 2012).

13. Chris Feudtner, MD, *Bittersweet: Diabetes, Insulin, and the Transformation of Illness* (Chapel Hill: The University of North Carolina Press, 2003), 52.

14. Michael Bliss, *The Making of Modern Medicine: Turning Points in the Treatment of Disease* (Chicago: The University of Chicago Press, 2011), 76.

15. Bliss, 76.

16. David O. Woodbury, "Please Save My Son" *Reader's Digest*, (volume 82, number 490, February, 1963), 157-162.

17. Robert Buynak, MD, *Dr. Buynak's 1-2-3 Diabetes Diet: A Step-by-Step Approach to Weight Loss without Gimmicks or Risks* (Alexandria, Virginia: American Diabetes Association, 2006), 85.

18. Beaser, 87,106

Health and Wellness Index

*"My son, pay attention to what I say. Listen closely to my words. Don't let them out of your sight. Keep them in your heart. They are life to those who find them. **They are health to your whole body"** (Proverbs 4:20-22). (Notice the principles or concepts taught in the proverbs listed.)

Blood glucose (BG)

Carbohydrates *"The wisdom of the prudent is to give thought to their ways, but the folly of fools is deception"* (Proverbs 14:8).

Portion Control *"When you sit down to eat with a ruler, look carefully at what's in front of you. Put a knife to your throat if you like to eat too much"* (Proverbs 23:1-2). *"If you find honey, eat just enough. If you eat too much of it, you will throw up . . . It isn't good for you to eat too much honey"* (Proverbs 25:16, 27). 168-170

Positive Self-talk *"Pleasant words are like honey. They are sweet to the spirit and bring healing to the body"* (Proverbs 16:24).

Record Keeping for Personal Health *"The prudent give thought to their steps"* (Proverbs 14:8). *"Be sure you know the condition of your flocks, give careful attention to your herds"* (Proverbs 27:23).

Self-control Development *"Like a city whose walls are broken through is a person who lacks self-control"* (Proverbs 25:28). *"A fool gives full vent to his anger, but a wise man keeps himself under control"* (Proverbs 29:11).

"In the house of the wise are stores of choice food and oil, but a foolish man devours all he has" (Proverb 21:20).
Realize God cares about you. Trust God, using His wisdom. ix, xvi, 39-40 *"the LORD gives wisdom, and from his mouth come knowledge and understanding. He holds victory in store for the upright, he is a shield to those whose walk is blameless, for **he guards the course of the just and protects the way of his faithful ones.** Then you will understand what is right and just and fair--every good path. For wisdom will enter your heart, and knowledge will be pleasant to your soul. **Discretion will protect you, and understanding will guard you** (Proverbs 2:6-11). "The fear of the LORD is the beginning of wisdom, and knowledge of the Holy One is understanding. **For through wisdom your days will be many, and years will be added to your life.** If you are wise, your wisdom will reward you . . ."* (Proverbs 9:10-12). *"**Trust in the LORD** with all your heart and lean not on your own understanding; in all your ways acknowledge him, and he will make your paths straight"* (Proverbs 3:5-6).
Purpose and meaning in life: Encourage others 12, 15-16, 93-97 *"Whoever oppresses the poor shows contempt for their Maker, but whoever is kind to the needy honors God"* (Proverbs 14:31). *"A generous person will prosper. Whoever refreshes others will be refreshed"* (Proverbs 11:25). *"A good person gives life to others; the wise person teaches others how to live"* (Proverbs 11:30).
To fail to plan is to plan to fail. Make the Best Decisions Ahead of Time: Be Diligent 184-185 *"The plans of the diligent lead to profit as surely as haste leads to poverty"* (Proverbs 21:5).
Diligence enhances self-control 188-189
Portion control enhances self-control 168-170
Gratitude and positive self-talk empowers persistent self-control 11-12, 78-80

house is built, and through understanding it is established; through knowledge its rooms are filled with rare and beautiful treasures" (Proverbs 24:3-4).

About the Author:

Ken Ellis is a fifty-three year survivor of diabetes, being diagnosed when he was in the first grade in 1960. For more than twenty-two years he has facilitated hospital and community diabetes support groups in several states, helping hundreds of people.

Ken has participated in the 50-year medalist research study at the world-renowned Joslin Diabetes Center, which is affiliated with Harvard Medical School in Boston. His accomplishment of diabetes management for more than fifty years has earned him the Joslin 50-Year Medal.

Education: Degree of Master of Science in Biblical Studies, Abilene Christian University, 1982
Contact: wisdomfordiabetes.org
email: ken@wisdomfordiabetes.org